NVLD and Developmental Visual-Spatial Disorder in Children

Jessica Broitman • Miranda Melcher
Amy Margolis • John M. Davis

NVLD and Developmental Visual-Spatial Disorder in Children

Clinical Guide to Assessment and Treatment

Springer

Jessica Broitman
International Control Mastery Therapy
Center (CMT)
Berkeley, CA, USA

Miranda Melcher
Department of Defense Studies
King's College London
London, UK

Amy Margolis
Brooklyn Learning Center
Columbia University Irving Medical Center
Brooklyn, NY, USA

John M. Davis
California State University, East Bay
Hayward, CA, USA

ISBN 978-3-030-56107-9 ISBN 978-3-030-56108-6 (eBook)
https://doi.org/10.1007/978-3-030-56108-6

This Springer imprint is published by the registered company Springer Nature Switzerland AG
The registered company address is: Gewerbestrasse 11, 6330 Cham, Switzerland

We dedicate this book to Brett and Moira, without whom this book would not have been written. We so appreciate that they trusted us to share their journey. Also, that they were willing to teach us what we needed to know, to help them become the amazing, successful adults they currently are. It is our hope that we are accurately taking the ideas we developed together in order to share them with the rest of our patients and colleagues to increase the knowledge and understanding of NVLD.

Foreword

Early in my career, I found Nonverbal Learning Disability (NVLD) to be a puzzle that frequently generated arguments but rarely yielded solutions. This book, from Drs. Broitman, Melcher, Margolis, and Davis, four experts who have given their careers to the evaluation and treatment of NVLD, does not spend its time quibbling about the puzzling pieces of NVLD but is instead explicitly focused on helping children to succeed—in school and in life. Its practical approach will make it a book that lives in the hands of clinicians and educators, rather than on a library shelf.

One of the more vexing challenges to those of us who evaluate and treat children is understanding what Nonverbal Learning Disability actually is. Without being included in our Diagnostic and Statistical Manual (DSM5), its diagnosis and definition can vary from clinician to clinician. Its name can also generate confusion, seemingly representing a double negative. Children with NVLD and their families often have to go on a diagnostic odyssey before they receive a diagnosis that is sometimes contradicted by the next clinician. Here, a rigorously refined definition is provided, together with a new name that describes the core symptoms of NVLD for what they are: Developmental Visual-Spatial Disorder (DVSD).

After providing a clear definition of what NVLD/DVSD is, the authors lay out how to evaluate and intervene with affected children. Importantly, I have never seen a child who has only ever received a diagnosis of NVLD. Before—or after—receiving this diagnosis, they often have been diagnosed with an anxiety disorder, Attention Deficit Hyperactivity Disorder (ADHD), a mood disorder, Autism Spectrum Disorder (ASD), Social (Pragmatic) Communication Disorder, or a non-specific learning disorder. Sometimes, these diagnoses are also correct—NVLD/DVSD seems to frequently co-occur with other conditions. Other times, an accurate diagnosis might have prevented or ameliorated school-related anxiety, social difficulties, or a depressive episode.

Here, the authors provide explicit guidance on how to differentiate NVLD/DVSD, even in the presence of other conditions. They even provide guidance for interpreting neuropsychology results from another provider to clarify a diagnosis. Importantly, they do not stop at defining NVLD/DVSD for clinicians but also describe explicitly how to explain and work with children and families who are trying to conceptualize their own experiences. I have found in my own clinical work that framing a child's difficulties in a brain-based conceptualization can be transformative, both for themselves and for their parents. Too often, children—and their parents—think that they lack intelligence, or effort, or moral fiber, instead of recognizing that they struggle with a specific domain of learning.

Educational intervention and treatment in NVLD/DVSD is an art form. These four authors are artists who have each approached it from different directions, whether as a psychotherapist, a teacher and tutor, a neuropsychologist, or a director of an educational program and clinic, and often multiple of the above. They synthesize these perspectives to provide straightforward guidance on approaches that have worked with children. This practical approach extends to how to work around challenges, how to engage and persist with homework, and specific interventions that target 11 categories of difficulty commonly seen in NVLD/DVSD.

I very much appreciate the practical—and humble—approach taken by the authors. Unfortunately, NVLD/DVSD is a few decades behind other conditions, like Autism Spectrum Disorder, which used to generate a similar diagnostic odyssey but are now the focus of evidence-based treatment approaches that are sometimes implemented as early as 18 months. Like in ASD, advocacy on the part of individuals and parents is pushing the field of NVLD/DVSD forward, as evidenced by the efforts of Dr. Lemle of The NVLD Project, who provides the Afterword for this text. I fully expect that this will just be the first edition of this text, with refinements to come as Drs. Broitman, Melcher, Margolis, Davis, and Lemle continue to push this field forward to better understand the early signs, refine the patterns of risk for co-occurring disorders, and develop evidence-based treatments for this important condition.

Jeremy Veenstra-VanderWeele
Ruane Professor of Child and Adolescent Psychiatry at Columbia University
New York, USA

Director of the Division of Child & Adolescent Psychiatry at
New York-Presbyterian/Morgan Stanley Children's Hospital, New York State
Psychiatric Institute (NYSPI)
Columbia University, New York, USA

Co-Director of both the NIMH T32 Postdoctoral Fellowship for Translational
Research in Child Psychiatric Disorders and the Whitaker Scholar Program in
Developmental Neuropsychiatry NYSPI/Columbia University Medical Center
New York, USA
Jeremy.Veenstra-VanderWeele@nyspi.columbia.edu

Acknowledgments

We would like to thank all of our patients and colleagues who, over the years, have shared their experiences and ideas with us and, in particular, Mariah DeSerisy, who provided crucial clinical insight. We also thank Gibor Basri, once again, for his assistance in editing.

Contents

About the Authors

Jessica Broitman is a psychoanalyst practicing in Berkeley since 1980. She began her career in Boulder, Colorado, in 1973. As a member of the Intensive Treatment Team of the Boulder Mental Health Center, she ran the Gordon Beyer project, which was one of the first residential treatment programs for young people with schizophrenia and bi-polar illness in the country. After moving to California in 1980, she became the Program Coordinator for the Creative Living Center, a day treatment program for adults with mental illness. During this time, she became involved with Joseph Weiss and Control Mastery Theory. She formalized the San Francisco Psychotherapy Research Group (http://sfprg.org) as a non-profit organization in 1993. She is President Emerita of SFPRG. She was instrumental in the initiation of SFPRG's Psychotherapy Training Center and Clinic, and served as the Executive Director for 15 years. In 2017 she helped create the International Control Mastery Therapy Center (CMT Center—https://cmtcenter.net) and currently serves as the President of the CMT Center. She frequently lectures on Weiss's Control Mastery Theory worldwide.

Dr. Broitman has been involved in researching and treating children with nonverbal learning disabilities and their families for more than 20 years. She is the co-author of *Nonverbal Learning Disabilities in Children: Bridging the Gap Between Science and Practice* (2011), and is the coeditor of *Treating NVLD in Children* (2013) as well as numerous chapters and articles. She is currently involved in several research projects concerning the treatment and understanding of NVLD and has a special interest in helping professionals and families understand and treat this disorder. She is available for consultations and can be reached at: drjess@comcast.net.

For more information on her work on NVLD see: Click on each book for more information.

For a half-hour video on NVLD featuring the authors, please see https://www.youtube.com/watch?v=vymdZUuB-T4&feature=youtu.be

Miranda Melcher is a teacher, security researcher, analyst, consultant, and author. She is currently pursuing her PhD on post-conflict military reconstruction at King's College London's Defence Studies Department with a planned graduation in May 2021. Her research identifies methods for integrating opposing forces into unified post-conflict security institutions. The aim of her PhD is to develop viable methods for rebuilding militaries and security institutions following civil wars. Miranda has also been a committed teacher and tutor for students ranging from 13 to 70 years of age, across a variety of subjects, focusing particularly on developing teaching practices around learning disabilities in both secondary and higher education. She is available for consultations and can be reached at: miranda.melcher@gmail.com

Amy E. Margolis is Assistant Professor of Medical Psychology at Columbia University Irving Medical Center and the Director of the Environment, Brain, and Behavior Lab. She has a doctorate in Applied Educational Psychology—School Psychology from Teacher's College and is trained as a clinical neuropsychologist with two decades of experience assessing and treating children with learning and attention disorders.

In 2013 she completed a T32 Fellowship in Translational Psychiatry at Columbia University and now conducts research as well as clinical practice. Dr. Margolis is an expert in human neuroimaging and focuses her learning disability research program on the brain basis of NonVerbal Learning Disability and the psychological factors that affect children with learning disorders such as anxiety and executive function problems.

Dr. Margolis is Principal or Co-investigator of several federally funded projects that use neuroimaging in longitudinal birth cohorts to study the effects of prenatal exposure to neurotoxicants on brain and behavior outcomes. Most recently she has served as the text reviser for the chapter on Specific Learning Disorder for DSM 5TR and is Co-chair of the ECHO (Environmental Influences on Children's Health Outcomes) National Neurodevelopment Working Group.

Recent publications from her lab include papers using functional MRI to study the neural correlates of NonVerbal Learning Disability as well as executive functions in reading disorder, anxiety in reading disorder, and the effects of prenatal exposure to commonly used flame retardants on the efficiency of the brain's reading network.

For more information on her work on NVLD see: https://www.ncbi.nlm.nih.gov/myncbi/amy.margolis.1/bibliography/public/; https://www.ebblab.com

And a webinar on NVLD at ADDitude Magazine:

https://www.additudemag.com/nonverbal-learning-disability-nvld-amy-margolis/

John M. Davis is currently a Full Professor and Chair of the Educational Psychology Department at California State University East Bay, and is teaching and supervising in their graduate programs. He is also in private practice in Lafayette, CA, where he specializes in the assessment of and consultation around learning disorders and disabilities in children, adolescents, and adults. He has also written and co-written over 40 articles and book chapters on a number of areas and co-authored 4 books, three of which are on learning disorders. He received his PhD from U.C. Berkeley in School Psychology, received postdoctoral training at U.C. Davis in Clinical/Family Psychology, and interned at the U.C. Davis Medical Center in Sacramento and at Children's Hospital in Oakland. He has worked in public schools, in a hospital-based Psychiatry Department at Kaiser in San Rafael, taught at a number of universities, and was Director of the Raskob Learning Institute in Oakland, CA, an assessment and remediation clinic and a day school for children with learning disorders. He can be reached at: davisjackm@aol.com or jack.davis@csueastbay.edu.

Chapter 1
Introduction

Nonverbal learning disability (NVLD) has been written about and discussed for roughly 60 years since it was named and described by Johnson and Myklebust (Johnson & Myklebust, 1967). Our recent work shows that 3–4% of the population of children in the United States are likely to have NVLD (Margolis et al. 2020). Nevertheless, there have been few empirically validated treatment options (Matte & Bolaski, 1998; Little, 1993; Davis and Broitman, 2016). *Treating NVLD in Children* (Broitman & Davis, 2013) provided practitioners with an understanding of the treatment needs of children with nonverbal learning disabilities and most importantly advocated for a team approach to treatment. This current book is intended to be a useful resource that follows up on that volume, as well as *NVLD in Children: Bridging the Gap Between Science and Practice* (Davis & Broitman, 2011). Although some books and articles begin to address the importance of a team approach for treating NVLD (Davis & Broitman, 2006, 2007, 2008; Forrest, 2004; Myklebust, 1975; Palombo, 2006; Tanguay, 2002), and some present treatments developed for classroom teachers and school-based professionals such as *Nonverbal Learning Disabilities and Their Clinical Subtypes: A Handbook for Parents and Professionals* (Mamen, 2006) and *Nonverbal Learning Disabilities at School, and Home* (Tanguay, 2002), there has yet to be a guide to a psychologically based specific treatment for the estimated 2.2 million to 2.9 million children and adolescents who may have a NVLD (Margolis et al. 2020).

Rourke's (1995) book on the *Syndrome of Nonverbal Learning Disabilities* offered a 15-point approach to treatment (amended by Tsatsanis & Rourke, 2003), most of which we would agree with from our clinical experience. He emphasized the need to utilize the child's strengths to remediate the areas of weakness and to plan for success using a realistic perspective to prepare the child with NVLD for adult life. Rourke (1995) differentiates the role of a psychologist from that of educators who have a particular curriculum to follow and teach. He states that the domain of the psychologist is as vast as the lifespan and that the child with NVLD very well may need help accruing all of life's social and survival skills.

J. Broitman et al., *NVLD and Developmental Visual-Spatial Disorder in Children*, https://doi.org/10.1007/978-3-030-56108-6_1

Like Rourke, we also think that the role of the psychologist is important in the treatment of NVLD, and this book outlines specifically how that can be accomplished using a team approach, working closely with patients; their families, schools, and tutors; and the many professionals that a child with NVLD will meet along their path. Accurate diagnostics, carefully chosen appropriate and individualized psychotherapeutic techniques, and interventions are required. We believe that mental health professionals have a unique and crucial role in helping the child with NVLD plan for and achieve success. We believe that sharing a transparent, psychologically minded approach offers the best chance of creating a successful collaboration with your patient and their family. In particular, when working with children with NVLD, practitioners must consider how the child's psychology (thoughts, feelings, and beliefs) affects their functioning and learning and how their experience is processed through their individual personality, psychology, culture, economic circumstances, and family dynamics. Utilizing these psychological organizing principles, this book describes how psychologists and other mental health professionals can best help their patients with NVLD.

1.1 Historical Overview of NVLD

The first mention of a potential NVLD-like syndrome was the Gerstmann syndrome in 1940, although he attributed it to a left hemisphere disorder. Gerstmann syndrome was characterized by difficulties in the areas of finger agnosia, right–left orientation, agraphia, and acalculia. Johnson and Myklebust noted "social perception disabilities" which they thought explained limitations in understanding nonverbal cues which impacted individuals' abilities to understand and respond to social interactions. They refined and renamed this syndrome nonverbal learning disability in 1967 (Johnson & Myklebust, 1967). In the 1970s, Rourke (1995) and his colleagues introduced a developmental neurological approach to studying learning disabilities and proposed the "white matter model" for the etiology of NVLD. Since then, there has been increased interest in understanding, defining, and treating NVLD. Our most recent consensus definition is presented in Chap. 3. Our latest understanding of the etiology of NVLD is presented in Chap. 4.

NVLD has no obvious visible effects on appearance that would identify its presence. It is primarily an invisible disability, which frequently confounds patients' access to early and accurate diagnosis and treatment. Adding to this, children with NVLD are often described as "precocious in verbal reasoning and language development," leading to them being seen as linguistically advanced rather than suffering from an impairment. As our methods for recognizing and diagnosing these children improve, we anticipate clarification and refinements of the profile of NVLD. We do, however, continue to see a unique pattern of strengths and challenges. Assets of children with NVLD often include early speech and vocabulary development, a relative strength in auditory/verbal rote memory, and strong attention to detail, and some would say an overfocusing on detail, often early reading skills, and often excellent spelling skills. Difficulties usually include problems in visual–spatial (core deficit) processing, organizational/executive function challenges, academic struggles (typically math), social functioning, and motor coordination issues. Associated difficulties include psychological issues and environmental sensitivities. Visual–spatial challenges reflect particular challenges with *visuospatial awareness* such as awareness of own body in space or personal space of others; *visuospatial construction* such as copying visually presented materials; *visuospatial working memory* such as holding spatial information in mind while simultaneously acting on that information; *visuospatial scanning/tracking* such as finding information on a page/poster or screen; *spatial estimation* such as judging distance, quantity, or time; *three-dimensional thinking* such as imagining how things will look when rotated; and *interpreting information presented pictorially* such as diagrams or maps.

Executive functioning challenges may include aspects of processing/regulation such as decision-making, planning, initiation, assigning priority, sequencing, emotional regulation, problem-solving, planning, impulse control, establishing goals, monitoring results of action, and self-correcting.

Social challenges can include difficulties with comprehending nonverbal communication, pragmatic language, adjusting to transitions, and coping with new or novel situations, along with some deficits in social judgment and social interaction.

Motor challenges may include gross or fine motor skills, poor coordination, balance problems, and difficulty learning gross motor skills such as riding a bike. In addition, difficulties with fine motor skills such as learning to tie one's shoes or graphomotor skills may also be present.

Academic difficulties, when they exist, are often in areas that require understanding or "reading" visual diagrams, such as in math, geography, and science. These subjects often require interpreting graphic material and integrating information into novel concepts or procedures. Difficulty with reading can also occur, not at the word-reading level but more often at the comprehension level. One hypothesis is that students with NVLD may have difficulty generating an internal visual image of what they are reading – seeing the story in their mind's eye. Developing written expression skills can also be hard for students with NVLD for many reasons, including difficulty organizing and sequencing ideas or motor difficulties that interfere with written expression (note: with respect to the range of gender identities, we will use the pronoun "they" when referring to students and patients throughout the manuscript).

Associated psychological difficulties or diagnoses may include attention deficit hyperactivity disorder (ADHD) and anxiety disorder. Other associated developmental disorders could be a specific learning disorder in math, developmental coordination disorder, autism spectrum disorder, and social communication disorder.

There have been many other observed and anecdotally reported associated features of NVLD including difficulty with pragmatic language, understanding whole–part relationships, contending with novelty, and environmental sensitivity to light brightness, screen color/brightness, temperature and humidity, sound, feel/touch of textures, and taste, to name a few (see Chap. 13 for an additional discussion of these). Once a consensus is reached for a clinical definition, further research will allow empirical tests of all of these areas of associated difficulties.

1.2 Book Overview

In this section, we describe the outline of the book beginning with Chap. 2: *Markers of NVLD Within a Developmental Framework*, wherein we introduce two of our patients, Brett and Moira, who will accompany you throughout the book, as we offer you a glimpse into the developmental signs of NVLD from infancy through high school.

In Chap. 3: *What Is a Nonverbal Learning Disability (NVLD)/Developmental Visual–Spatial Disorder* we suggest a new definition for *nonverbal learning disorders (NVLD)*. We report on the current project to create a new name/definition for NVLD and our work to gain inclusion in the *Diagnostic and Statistical Manual (DSM)*. This work is being done by a consortium led by Prudence W. Fisher, PhD, Division of Child and Adolescent Psychiatry, Columbia University College of Physicians and Surgeons, and NVLD global experts: Drs. Amy Margolis Jessica Broitman, Joseph Casey, John (Jack) M. Davis, Jodene Goldenring Fine, Irene Mammarella, M. Douglas Ris, and Margaret Semrud-Clikeman, and members of The NVLD Project's Board of Directors and Advisory Board.

In Chap. 4, *The Etiology and Pathophysiology of NVLD*, we discuss our most recent understanding of these issues. We also consider common comorbidities with NVLD and their relevance for treatment considerations.

In Chap. 5, *The Initial Contact and the Intake Process*, we lay out the specific steps one must take to determine what treatment and/or assessment is needed.

In Chap. 6, *A Screening and Diagnostic Assessment for NVLD*, we lay out the assessment process, which is critical for the diagnosis of NVLD, and address how you present the results to the family and/or patient with NVLD.

In Chap. 7, *Reading and Interpreting a Neuropsychological Assessment Report*, we discuss how to interpret and read the results of an assessment report. We present the common composition of a test report. We offer a guide to the structure and types of scores utilized in the report and how to use the data and results to read and understand a test report. Lastly, we offer a "how to" for professionals to make provisional diagnosis of NVLD using prior documentation when new testing is not available.

In Chap. 8, *The Need for Treatment*, we present our current understanding regarding the need for early and specific intervention.

In Chap. 9, *Working with a Consistent Psychological Theory*, we discuss the importance of working from a shared theoretical orientation. This chapter addresses how all of the professionals on the team must be well versed in understanding the underlying psychological issues that are presented when someone has NVLD. A model theory, Weiss' control mastery theory (CMT), is presented.

In Chap. 10, *Creating a Treatment Plan and Team*, we offer a step-by-step guide to creating your team and treatment plan using the diagnostic information at hand.

In Chap. 11, *Working with Your Patient's Family*, we offer specific tips for helping families navigate the complexity of family dynamics.

In Chap. 12, *Learning from Our Patients*, we offer techniques to work with our patients to tailor their treatment to their specific needs.

In Chap. 13, *Choosing What to Work On First in Therapy/Tutoring*, we consider the timing of interventions. This chapter helps you navigate how to decide which issues to address, in what order, including how to break them down and create a plan for each specific problem your patient faces.

In Chap. 14, *The Brooklyn Learning Center Model*, we describe a model for psychological treatment for NVLD that incorporates academic tutoring and cognitive remediation, and we offer specific strategies for working with students with NVLD.

In Chap. 15, *Specific Interventions*, we offer guidelines and possible interventions to consider in the categories of visual–spatial, executive functioning, academics, social/emotional challenges, motor coordination, and sensory issues.

And lastly in Chap. 16, *Conclusions*, we offer our closing thoughts. The appendices include copies of our forms and checklists for you to use. Join us now to meet Brett and Moira, the stars of this book, in Chap. 2.

References

Broitman, J., & Davis, J. M. (2013). *Treating NVLD in children: Professional collaborations for positive outcomes*. New York: Springer.

Davis, J., & Broitman, J. (2006). A brief overview of nonverbal learning disorders. *The Educational Therapist, 27*(3), 5–10.

Davis, J., & Broitman, J. (2007). Nonverbal learning disabilities: Models of proposed subtypes, part II. *The Educational Therapist, 27*(4), 5–10.

Davis, J., & Broitman, J. (2008). *Nonverbal learning disabilities: Diagnosis and history*. Hawaii: Paper presented at the International Neuropsychological Society Annual Convention.

Davis, J., & Broitman, J. (2011). *Nonverbal learning disabilities in children: Bridging the gap between science and practice*. New York: Springer Publications.

Davis, J., & Broitman, J. (2016). *Team collaborations for the best-practice treatment of NVLD across three systems: School. Hospital and family based*. In B. Rissman (Ed.), *Medical and educational perspectives on NVLD in children and young adults*. Hershey, PA: IGI Global.

Forrest, B. (2004). The utility of math difficulties, internalized psychopathology, and visual spatial deficits to identify children with the nonverbal learning disability syndrome: Evidence for a visual-spatial disability. *Child Neuropsychology, 10*(2), 129–146. https://doi.org/10.1080/09297040490911131.

Johnson, D. J., & Myklebust, H. R. (1967). *Learning disabilities: Educational principles and practices*. New York: Grune & Stratton.

Little, S. S. (1993). Nonverbal learning disabilities and socioemotional functioning: A review of recent literature. *Journal of Learning Disabilities, 26*, 653–665.

Mamen, M. (2006). *Nonverbal learning disabilities and their clinical subtypes: A handbook for parents and professionals*. Nepean, ON: Centrepointe Professional Services.

Margolis, A. E., Broitman, J., Davis, J. M., Alexander, L., Hamilton, A., Liao, Z., et al. (2020). Estimated prevalence of nonverbal learning disability among north American children and adolescents. *JAMA Network Open, 3*(4), e202551. https://doi.org/10.1001/jamanetworkopen.2020.2551.

Matte, R. R., & Bolaski, J. A. (1998). Nonverbal learning disabilities: An overview. *Intervention in School and Clinic, 34*(1), 39–43.

Myklebust, H. R. (1975). Nonverbal learning disabilities: Assessment and intervention. In H. R. Myklebust (Ed.), *Progress in learning disabilities* (Vol. III, pp. 85–121). New York: Grune & Stratton.

Palombo, J. (2006). *Nonverbal learning disabilities: A clinical perspective.* New York: W.W. Norton.

Rourke, B. P. (1995). The NLD syndrome and the white matter model. In B. P. Rourke (Ed.), *Syndrome of nonverbal learning disabilities: Neurodevelopmental manifestations* (pp. 1–27). New York: Guilford Press.

Tanguay, P. B. (2002). *Nonverbal learning disabilities at school.* London: Jessica Kingsley, Publishers.

Tsatsanis and Rourke. (2003). *Syndrome of nonverbal learning disabilities: Effects on learning.* In A. H. Fine & R. A. Kotkin (Eds.), *Therapist's guide to learning and attention disorders.* Amsterdam: Elsevier.

Chapter 2
Markers of NVLD Within a Developmental Framework

We first must stress that no two children with NVLD look exactly the same or fit the same developmental pattern (Rourke, 1995). With possible challenges in four major areas (executive functions, social, academic, and motor coordination) in conjunction with a spatial deficit, people with NVLD can end up presenting with very different clinical pictures, as outlined in the previous chapter.

In many cases, children are first identified as having NVLD in the third or fourth grade when difficulties with math and/or reading comprehension emerge. If not identified then, they can be identified later, even in high school or college, when difficulties with complex math or written expression can emerge. Moreover, individuals with NVLD struggle in school with issues that are not strictly academic (related to impairment in executive function, motor, social difficulties), and thus, they can go without assessment or intervention for long periods of time even though they are struggling. Advanced verbal skills in children with NVLD often compound this phenomenon. Their strong verbal skills can be a source of confusion for the adults around them, who can misunderstand their challenges, attributing them incorrectly to not trying hard enough or not paying attention.

Individuals with NVLD are also known for getting along very well with adults, and this fact may delay recognition that they are having social problems. This likely happens when adults provide scaffolding for children with NVLD without even realizing they are doing so. For example, adults may fill in missing transitions during a conversation or support the idiosyncratic interests that children with NVLD may have. We have also seen differences in presentations between girls and boys, with girls sometimes being better able to manage their social challenges.

In the next section, we offer some early indicators that can help identify the needs of children with NVLD. We introduce two of our patients, *Brett and Moira* (names and details altered to protect patients' privacy). Anecdotes from their lives will be used throughout the book to illustrate some of the differences in profiles. Brett was formally diagnosed with NVLD in fourth grade, while Moira did not receive a diagnosis of NVLD until her sophomore year of college.

J. Broitman et al., *NVLD and Developmental Visual-Spatial Disorder in Children*, https://doi.org/10.1007/978-3-030-56108-6_2

2.1 Infancy and Preschool Signs

We hypothesize that the precursors of the NVLD subtypes that are most frequently seen during this period will include motor challenges, as this is frequently the first major developmental challenge for children with NVLD. Most parents, however, report very early language acquisition for children with NVLD. *Brett, for example, could speak in full sentences by 8 months of age and count to 10 (by ones) in four languages by age 2. However, when asked to count how many objects were in front of him, he had no idea of what a number actually was and couldn't reply. He never crawled, but began to walk within the expected range at 1 year of age. He initiated little exploration or engagement and manipulation of his environment. As mentioned earlier, his parents joked that they wasted their money babyproofing their home in anticipation of normal exploration, yet Brett never opened a cupboard or tried to stick anything into a plug. His reading was also delayed till late kindergarten. He loved watching the same TV shows (Barney) over and over and over again, with little interest in anything new or novel.*

He was very uncomfortable with any type of parental separation or transition, without any understandable cause. His preschool was a highly respected lab school with an innovative format with children arranging their own schedule of activities according to their interests. Many educators rotated in and out throughout the week to offer exciting options to explore. Brett spent most of his time there asking who was going to teach today and when could he go home. Needless to say, this experimental program didn't last, and although his parents were mystified regarding the cause, he was moved to a more traditional preschool that had significantly less stimulation and his anxiety lessened.

Moira on the other hand was on the slightly earlier side for achieving these developmental milestones. She began both talking and walking entirely within the normal range. She learned to read just before kindergarten. She never had any issues with fine or gross motor control. She started going to ballet class at age 4 and tennis at age 6.

In normal development as described by Piaget (Inhelder & Piaget, 1964), the first stage of development is the sensorimotor stage, whereby much of learning is about the child's interactions with their environment and on a sensory level. However, children with NVLD often have developmental delays leading to less exposure to sensorimotor learning (Davis & Broitman, 2011). As Rourke (1995) suggests, when describing children with NVLD, "these children (often) remain essentially sedentary, exploring the world not through vision or locomotion, but rather through receiving verbal answers to questions posed about the immediate environment" (p. 8). The disparity between their language development, especially vocabulary, and the delays in motor development in the child is most notable in the early years (Davis & Broitman, 2011).

For infants and toddlers, these initial concerns are most often problems with sensory and motor processing, sensitivity to light or loud noises, and difficulty with fine and gross motor skills and might promote one to consult with a pediatrician to rule out other potential neurological causes. However, as early development is often inconsistent and individual, professionals often take a wait-and-see attitude during these years, assuming the delay is not diagnostic and that the child will overcome any delays without intervention.

Anecdotal reports from parents of children with NVLD often state that during infancy their child would sit and point at an object, saying what they wanted rather than crawling toward it. Many of these children do not use typical toddler toys or enjoy coloring or drawing. They are usually disinterested in or unable to put puzzles together (Johnson, 1987). They are often clumsy and slower to develop gross and fine motor skills needed to feed themselves, brush their hair, and dress themselves. Group activities and play are mystifying to our children with NVLD as the rules are ever changing and communicated nonverbally. They can display environmental sensitivity to textures, foods, sound, and light. *Both Brett and Moira have expressed issues with "mushy foods," and Brett has a variety of sound sensitivities.*

Parents additionally report less than expected eye contact and mirroring. *Both Brett and Moira had to be taught to look directly at people. Moira still struggles with this and has spoken of coming up with tricks to make it look like she is looking at others on Zoom.* Parents are often confused when their extremely verbal child is not developing consistently across developmental lines. They may create unwarranted and inaccurate expectations, based upon inappropriate assumptions about their child's superior language development. Problems for the child can become exacerbated when poor motor and spatial development can disappoint and confound the parents. Early sensorimotor exploration is important in the child's development, since learning depends upon the interaction of the child with the environment (Piaget, 1972). Although children with NVLD are interacting with their environment, their interactions are more often verbal and observational and less frequently motoric and spatial, altering their developmental trajectory. It is likely that less interaction and practice exploring the environment with the body may lead to less efficiency in motor skills compared to children with many more hours of practice. In turn, as they grow older, children with less confidence in their motor skills may be less inclined to engage in activities demanding it, further reducing their skill growth and development.

2.2 Early Schooling Signs

Kindergarten teachers may be the first to notice and call out problems in fine motor skills in a child with NVLD. These children have failed to "simply catch up" to their developing peers. We hypothesize that the subtypes that emerge most frequently during this period all include motor challenges: visual–spatial and motor/math deficits and visual–spatial and motor/social. The child may struggle more than his peers with items such as puzzles, scissors, crayons, or pencils. *Both Moira and Brett had difficulty learning to tie their shoes, and both still don't do it the way everyone else does.* As demands for writing and drawing increase in the classroom, the teacher may notice immaturity in children with NVLD compared to typically developing peers. *Brett, for example, could not read or write his name. He dealt with this at a screening interview for elementary school by telling the teacher who asked him to do so that "I haven't decided whether to come here yet, so I'd like to do the tour first." They forgot to ask him again later.* The teacher may turn to an occupational therapist (OT) for consultation and guidance as was the case for *Brett. His drawings seemed immature with no awareness of line. This led to an evaluation by the learning specialist at his school, in kindergarten. Her findings were positive for a visual/perceptual disability and a motor coordination problem. He was referred for a physical therapy evaluation which was positive for a sensory motor issue, and he was diagnosed with "dyspraxia" which was described to him as: "his muscles were having trouble hearing what his brain wanted him to do. We are going to train your muscles to get the messages better so you could have more fun and control." He was referred to occupational therapy and had 4 years of 2x/week treatment. Brett said "I would look at monkey bars and jump ropes and see everybody around me using them with ease and pleasure. Gross motor skills (throwing a ball, riding a bike, etc.) were delayed and difficult. For me, such activities were neither easy nor pleasurable. I would attempt them and my body would be unable to navigate them." To this day, he struggles with cartwheels! On the other hand, he developed a successful but idiosyncratic way of drawing by third grade. He would draw pictures of people dressed in costumes that were quite good, but he would start at the feet.*

Occupational therapists (OT) generally provide a physical assessment of gross and fine motor coordination, visual motor integration (VMI), visual and sensory processing, and written expression skills. They develop an OT treatment plan and interventions with follow-up evaluations. Sensory integration therapy (Ayres, 1994) might be offered to treat what the OT views as a sensory integration disability, although this is still considered a somewhat controversial intervention. If the child's issues are in the mild to moderate range, this may be all that is offered. Anecdotally, we find that many of our patients with NVLD describe environmental sensitivities (with the causes unknown) from an early age. *Moira remembers evidence early on of aversions of touching dirty things (sand, dirt, grass, etc.) and light sensitivity; she did not enjoy being outside at all.*

Sometimes children with NVLD may be referred for help with non-phonological reading difficulties (Pennington, 1991), but intervention may be premature. Rourke (1995) notes that these difficulties may well be developmental for children with NVLD, and most children with NVLD develop basic reading skills without intervention. Thompson (1997) hypothesized that reading was a new task for our children, and all novelty is initially problematic. As children with NVLD are often helped with clear rules, Martin (2007) suggests that programs designed for children with dyslexia can be useful for our children as they rely heavily on teaching rules.

However, Griffin and Gresham (2002) theorize that these reading problems are often associated with difficulties in visual processing problems, like tracking. Tracking refers to the ability of the child to stay on the correct line of reading or math without veering off course creating confusion and extra time for the student to reorient oneself. They further theorize that these problems are due to visual–spatial processing difficulties and claim that children with NVLD frequently require tracking training with as many as 30% needing to be *retrained* in order to read fluently. He suggests performing a thorough optometric examination that includes an assessment of visual tracking. *Brett was referred to an optometry clinic for tracking training with Dr. Grisham, a developmental optometrist, which consisted of 6 months of daily eye exercises which would need to be repeated at age 14.*

Often children with NVLD develop early math difficulties, although some use their verbal memory strengths to help them compensate through the early grades and occasionally beyond. Estimation, understanding concepts, lining up numbers correctly on a page, and recognizing the correct mathematical signs can be problematic. These difficulties are often viewed only as difficulty with math. We hypothesize that in girls with good classroom behavior (rule following) and adequate social standing (parents make playdates for children, all children are invited to all birthday parties, etc.), the math problems may be ignored or overlooked, possibly due to gender stereotyping.

If they have not emerged earlier in preschool, during this early elementary period, concerns may begin to develop about social perception and pragmatic language development as so much of parametric speech is conveyed through nonverbal means. They often rely on literal and concrete interpretations of words (Martin, 2007). It is often difficult for them to recognize and understand jokes, sarcasm, or teasing. Further, boys and girls with NVLD can present with clinical signs of anxiety, depression, attention problems, obsessional preoccupations, and self-esteem problems (Palombo & Berenberg, 1999), and a study by Mooney, Newberry, and Kurtz (2006) found that 41% of students with NVLD were misdiagnosed as having behavioral problems.

The mechanism through which the spatial deficits that characterize NVLD affect social interactions remains understudied. Spatial deficits may give rise to social difficulties through reduced processing capacities, for example, difficulty with processing facial expressions and social signals, managing executive functions that are inherent in social interactions, or novel problem-solving to name a few. Social difficulties could instead arise from underlying spatial processing deficits through reduced interaction with peers due to their environmental sensitivities and sensorimotor issues (Hale & Fiorello, 2004). We do know that students with NVLD often interact more successfully with adults than with their peers. Possibly adults are able to provide support for these students without conscious awareness of the scaffolding they provide. *Brett's family described him as very uncomfortable at birthday parties or gymnastics classes as he seemed overstimulated and anxious. Moira at age 5 asked her parents to not have to attend birthday parties, a request that was granted to Moira's relief.* Clearly further research is required to test behavioral pathways through which spatial deficits yield social difficulties.

With difficulties communicating in the social arena, especially with pragmatic language problems, the child with NVLD next often encounters a speech and language therapist. Speech and language therapists explore the communicative characteristics associated with NVLD specifically language form: phonology, morphology, syntax, semantics, and pragmatics and if relevant examine areas of overlap with other diagnostic categories, in particular high-functioning autism (HFA). During earlier stages, these children might have been seen for articulation issues connected with poor oral–motor functions, while in early elementary school, they are more likely seen for pragmatic language difficulties in social discourse.

Children with NVLD often do not use appropriate vocal intonations. They might speak in a flat monotone or with a singsong voice. It can be difficult to read their mood from their facial expressions, and they may seem wooden and constricted (Palombo & Berenberg, 1999). In speech and language nomenclature, these issues are often called semantic–pragmatic disabilities (Volden, 2004). Their fluent, sophisticated language may mislead conversational partners into assuming that the speaker with NVLD has equally sophisticated social comprehension. Coupled with difficulties in taking appropriate conversational turns, repairing communication breakdowns, maintaining conversational topics, and navigating social situations, these children can experience repeated failure and rejection in school and in the wider community. These children often "slip through the cracks" in terms of service provision. It is believed to bode well for youngsters if these issues are identified early, and intervention begins before the child falls behind allowing secondary features, especially anxiety, to develop (Palombo & Berenberg, 1999). *Looking back at videos, even as a baby, Moira seemed incredibly literal, with robotic tone and lack of variance in facial expressions, and as a young adult, she still struggles with facial expressions and vocal intonations.*

Even though children with these processing difficulties may struggle and become frustrated by math or aspects of written expression, they tend not to be referred yet to special educators because they perform "well enough." Their superior verbal skills often cause educators and parents to assume that their difficulties arise from insufficient effort or difficulty paying attention. Some are even considered "gifted" given their precocious language development. Rourke (1995) wrote that young children with these symptoms are often misdiagnosed with ADHD or seen as having only ADHD. Unfortunately such missed diagnoses can lead to a host of self-esteem problems and psychological issues, particularly when appropriate interventions are then not available. *In Moira's case, it is clear that her superior intellect and verbal mediation talents enabled her to avoid diagnosis until college, leading to a host of secondary psychological issues.*

2.3 Later Elementary and Middle School Signs

As academic subjects become more abstract, and more independent work is expected, children with NVLD often begin to experience greater difficulties. Executive function demands increase, and children with NVLD and their parents report that they have notable difficulty with tasks requiring executive functions such as getting started on tasks (initiation), keeping track of multiple sets of information (set shifting), inhibiting a common response in favor of a more challenging response (inhibitory control), problems keeping track of their papers (organization), keeping track of progress toward a goal (self-monitoring), developing a strategy to try different approach to a task (cognitive flexibility), and shifting to a different task (transition).

As the school years progress, even more difficulties with reading comprehension, math, and writing emerge, which are likely often driven by deficits in executive functions and attention capacity. Usually the teacher notices difficulties in school-related performance and attributes these difficulties to inattention or executive dysfunction, which is then communicated to the family. Social, emotional, and behavioral difficulties may have also become more pronounced, and referrals are often made to physicians such as general pediatricians, behavioral pediatricians, child and adolescent psychiatrists, and pediatric neurologists. Throughout all of this, there is often little notice or mention of a visual–spatial deficit, because we have not trained teachers and physicians to look for these deficits.

Lipton (2013) suggests that medications might be considered useful for dealing with specific symptoms and associated conditions rather than to the primary problem of a visual–spatial deficit (for more information, see Chap. 6, "The Physician's Role in Treating NVLD in Broitman and Davis Treating NVLD in Children"). We hypothesize that the subtypes most frequently seen during this period will be the visual–spatial and math executive function deficits or visual–spatial and math/social deficits or the more compounding visual–spatial–math, social, and executive function profile.

Educational therapists might become involved during this period. They can offer specific tutoring as well as make recommendations to the schools for the best practice teaching methods for children with NVLD when they have reading comprehension and written expression challenges. Educational therapists can specifically address how to teach math to children who have NVLD, helping them to learn the vocabulary of mathematics, the procedures of mathematics, and the major concepts of mathematics.

Neuropsychologists and school psychologists can also help put in place testing accommodations and classroom curriculum modifications when appropriate. To address students' deficits in attention and executive functioning that result in unequal access to standardized tests and in-class assignments, they can request that students receive 50% extra time on all tests, etc. Given students' difficulty with novelty, they might ask that the student be allowed to take high-stakes exams at their home school with which they are familiar, or if not possible testing should be provided a separate location to minimize distractions. Preferential seating is often suggested along with explicit study guides, sample problems or reminders, and modified test questions.

Our children's level of challenge appears to be connected to how high their verbal intelligence is and how significant the visual–spatial deficit is. The higher their verbal intelligence, the more successfully they seem to be able to mediate their visual–spatial challenges. *Moira, for example, had an extremely high verbal intelligence at the 99th %, which was 34 standard score points above her performance intelligence (which was in the average range). She would say that she always loved school and the idea of school and learning. Her academic issues did not become apparent until later in high school and college. Math was initially fun and easy, at least the algebra her dad taught her at home, which she liked much more than the easy geometric math at school. Both Brett and Moira also remember that learning to read analog clocks was difficult, which is another area subject to spatial processing challenges.*

Math concepts increasingly rely on spatial awareness rather than rote memorization, and frequently children with NVLD have notable trouble learning these spatially based concepts. Number lines, place values, decimals, operational signs, whole–part relationships, ratios, percents, and estimations all present notable challenges. Educational therapists might become involved during this period to specifically address how to work on math with children who have NVLD. Often the educational therapist must describe how to learn the vocabulary of mathematics, the procedures of mathematics, and the major concepts of mathematics. Depending on the level of difficulty, the student may or may not be referred for a psychoeducational or neuropsychological evaluation at this time. *In Brett's case by fourth grade, it was apparent that the "problem" was more than simple dyspraxia. His math skills were significantly below grade level and his thinking appeared "unique." A referral was made for a full neuropsychology assessment which confirmed a 40-standard score point discrepancy between VIQ and PIQ, along with other visual–spatial, executive function, social, and motor difficulties. This resulted in a diagnosis of atypical NVLD which was described to him as "he saw things differently than most people and had his own unique way of understanding things."*

His family knew that he had been aware of this and had come up with his own ways of coping. Unfortunately some of them took a lot of effort and interfered with how easy it was to learn things. Some of the things he did got him into trouble with friends at school (like talking to himself to decompress). Together they were going to sort it out and figure out how to help him. His family offered a lot of apologies as they had thought that he was not trying. This diagnosis led to the addition of weekly therapy with a neuropsychologist to work on executive functions and math and sessions with a physical trainer.

Brett said: "My team has been both large and small depending on my developmental needs. In the beginning I saw someone almost every day, and by the end I was basically just seeing a single neuropsychologist. By the end of my time with this man, I was prepared to teach myself. The thing that he got more than anyone else was the importance of breaking down an assignment into individualized steps. My learning specialist realized that the more crowded a page was, the harder it was for me to see essential information. We spent a lot of time breaking down an assignment into chunks of essential information and tackling them one by one. Because NVLD has an organizational deficit, it was important for me to have someone teach me how to break down tasks into manageable chunks. He would literally go over each and every step of something repeatedly till I knew how to replicate it. The best way I can describe what he did is say that he made space for me to learn. He took what was too convoluted and congested for me and helped give it breathing room so I could digest it. He called it 'reducing cognitive overload'."

Given the assessment data, helping professional observations, and discussions with Brett and his parents, the following accommodations were also arranged to reduce stress and enhance academic functioning:

(1) *Preferential registration to classes with teachers who are sensitive to LD issues (very clear about expectations and assignments – understands that materials may not get to school in a timely manner and a willingness to modify assignments that emphasize visual–spatial issues, or sequential multistep processes to allow him to show mastery, does not penalize unduly for small errors or reversals and supports thinking and creativity) to help reduce stress and to maintain Brett's self-esteem.*
(2) *Because he was a visually slower processor: longer test time, in a distraction-free environment, a recorder for bubble tests, and revised spacing on tests when needed to reduce the visual–spatial components of the test.*
(3) *Due to executive function challenges, it was requested that homework assignments listed on the web, faxed, or e-mailed home in order to reduce the pressure to get the assignment off the board at the same time as well as needing to transition to another class in another classroom.*
(4) *PE reassigned to appropriate activities as his motor coordination issues prevented successfully participating in the more typical activities of PE.*
(5) *Permission to dictate to parents or helper or record long assignments and use of a laptop to overcome his poor and slow handwriting.*
(6) *Copies of class notes to be made available in order to allow him to just listen and take in the material without the additional burden to write down what he was hearing which would be a slow labor-intensive process for him.*
(7) *Permit the use of a calculator due to his difficulty with math concepts and modifications of visually spatially based assignments (graphs/charts).*

Increasing social skills demands end up creating significant additional stress and frustration that can elevate anxiety which also makes academic progress difficult. At this point, academically oriented professionals often become involved in the lives of children with NVLD. Teachers become alarmed and mention their concerns at parent conferences. *Brett's social problems had continued, and he was socially isolated, often found wandering around talking to himself in the schoolyard. Penny, one of our patients, actually walked around talking to herself and her 52 imaginary friends. Moira remembers kind of having friends, but says she really didn't want them. She says she loved her Playmobil and lining up her dolls and found other kids to be loud and just not very interesting. She read a lot and got very annoyed when she wasn't allowed to read. Both Brett's and Moira's parents remember them asking to not go to birthday parties and not noticing or feeling left out when everyone else went to parties or played team sports.*

They both were bullied in school and preferred to spend lunch break alone or with a teacher than with peers. Moira describes looking for "the darkest shadiest corner of the field walking in patterns and talking to myself about characters in books I was reading and going to ballet class after school. Being in Girl Scouts was deeply irritating, something I refused to be subtle about to my mom's dismay. Generally, I preferred my social interactions limited, 1:1, quiet, and highly structured." Additionally, she recalled that "Being in the school musical (it was mandatory) was a hell of noise and repetition and everyone was slow – I don't like being center stage or acting; it feels like putting on a plastic uncomfortable mask, to make my face do things I'm not feeling. My performance was (now) hilariously robotic, the makeup was horrific on my skin, the bright lights glaring, and my general attitude was 'get me out of here'."

Moira began complaining out loud about light sensitivity in the fourth grade, specifically that the classroom lights were too bright. She was taken to get her eyes checked and given glasses despite the fact she didn't have vision issues. It took years to correctly understand the problem and to get dark glasses. Instead, every time she complained about bright lights (which was by her report, at least a few times a school year from fourth grade on), she was taken for a vision test. This was not correctly managed until adulthood. She was extremely sensitive to heat and sunburn, but the heat issue was generally overlooked due to a family of pale skin, and in the summer, she was able to stay in the shade or the pool which was fine due to low humidity.

Parents often reach out to ask for help for their children during this period, and public or private school wheels are set in motion. Student Study Team (SST) meetings are called or Individualized Educational Plans (IEP) are developed, the latter based upon psychoeducational evaluations in order to develop appropriate interventions (Hale & Fiorello, 2004; Telzrow & Bonar, 2002). Providing the best assistance for the student can become problematic because so much depends upon who gets involved and what they already know about NVLD. The child's parents also need to educate themselves to become more knowledgeable as they will become increasingly involved in their child's treatment team.

Helpful books for parents include Sue Thompson's *The Source for Nonverbal Learning Disorders* (1997); Pamela Tanguay's *Nonverbal Learning Disabilities at Home* (2001) or *Nonverbal Learning Disabilities at School* (2002); Kathy Allen's *Star Shaped Pegs, Square Holes: Nonverbal Learning Disabilities and the Growing Up Years* (1998); and Rondalyn Whitney's *The Nonverbal Learning Disability Guide for Teachers, Parents, Employers, and Therapists* (2000). The SST or IEP teams could advise them to join the Nonverbal Learning Disabilities Association (www.nlda.org) or to become familiar with websites such as The NVLD Project's https://nvld.org, Judy Lewis's www.nldline.com, Pam Tanguay's www.NLDontheweb.org, or the Charles Schwab website, www.schwablearning.org. More detailed information related to working with families is provided in a later chapter.

2.3.1 High School Signs

The high school experience can provide multiple challenges for patients with NVLD. Secondary symptoms such as poor self-esteem, anxiety, and sadness which can lead to depression may become apparent. Anxiety, in particular, is a frequent presenting complaint for children with NVLD. Children who have significant problems reading the visual/nonverbal cues which make up to 75% of communication (Mehrabian, 1971) often have a hard time making sense of what is happening in their environment. Anxiety can be a natural response to living in a confusing place where you understand neither what is happening nor what may happen. We hypothesize that the subtypes most frequently seen to emerge during this period are the visual–spatial and social/math deficits, visual–spatial and social deficits/executive functions, and their combination (visual–spatial + social + math + executive functions), potentially yielding more severe presentations. These newly recognized symptoms might once again prompt a referral to a physician to consider medications. Lipton (2013) finds that children with anxiety and mood disorders may be successfully treated with selective serotonin reuptake inhibitors (SSRIs).

Most high school environments are less structured than elementary and middle schools, with multiple classrooms and campuses, with many more teachers each with differing expectations, covering different subjects, lockers, and books to keep track of and be sure to have when needed in the correct location. So many parents say they found it simpler (if possible) to get the school to provide, borrow, or buy two sets of all textbooks one for home and one for school to avoid the continual driving back to one location or the other to get the needed book! *Brett's therapist explained to his somewhat shocked parents that there were actually 60 procedural steps required to correctly copy down a homework assignment and return it completed the next day. Teachers frequently complain that their students are late to class, forget their work, and are unable to complete tasks in the expected time limits. Moira on the other hand was always organized and never needed any help with homework until college. Instead her difficulties lay in the social–emotional realm.*

During high school, social skills can become a source of even greater concern, as social stresses, such as the demands of dating, are increased. *Moira found friendships complicated and unpredictable, finding herself blindsided by unexpected rants and responses she didn't understand. She said that she generally felt there was a massive disconnect between her and everyone else, that she had to wear "masks" all the time, and that something was not right. Brett's high school choice turned out to offer a much needed reprise from his extremely difficult middle school. He attended a very small, very structured school targeting bright children with some learning or developmental differences. He formed friendships and socialized for the first time. He says he found learning how to be socially successful complicated; he says he watched a lot of exaggerated situational comedies which made certain dynamics clearer than they might have been in real life.*

Brett describes feeling like there was an unwritten rule book that you need to study in terms of how far to stand away from people and when to make eye contact and learned that the rules were less concrete than he previously thought. He says: "I learned that if you watch and listen to other people, they will show you how they want to be interacted with. Everyone learns how to interact from their environment; it just took me longer." He warns of feeling like he had to fake certain kinds of interactions and join clubs, learn how to throw parties, etc. for the sake of guaranteeing contact with others. "I spent a lot of energy in my early teen years becoming friends with people I didn't even like just because they were willing to talk to me, putting a lot of effort into managing a façade in order to just have any kind of social life. It took me a long time to be able to choose who I actually wanted to be friends with and to understand that I didn't have to fake social interactions. I could be true to who I was and do the things I wanted to do" (see Broitman and Davis (2013), Treating NVLD in Children, Chap. 16, for more of Brett's story).

Advanced math and sciences will also be more challenging, requiring our children to explain hypothesis, theories, and abstract concepts. Lab work is impacted by challenges with fine motor skill and difficulty following procedural instruction. Our patients can no longer rely on their excellent rote memories. Math now relies heavily on visual–spatial competencies asking for judgments on dimension, size, and proportion in a language Martin (2007) calls "gibberish" for children with NVLD. *Moira's family had moved by this time to a much larger city, with bad pollution and serious humidity. She had begun to find certain topics in math hard, mainly matrices, calculus graphs, and statistics, but was still an overall happy B student in math with no particular issues with math or negative reports from any teachers.* Complex and advanced written expression assignments and advanced reading skills can present major challenges in the upper grades.

Moira was surprised to be plagued by a very weird record in what had always been her strongest subjects, History, Economics, and English which no one could figure out. In particular, writing problems emerged wherein she had difficulty translating her brilliant expansive ideas into clear coherent, concise essays. These challenges are often referred to as salience determination and can be found in the writings of Mel Levine (2002). Essentially, issues with salience determination mean that a student can learn a lot of information about the topic, but has trouble figuring out the relative importance of these ideas and their relative relevance. This therefore leads to essays that contain accurate information, but may be disorganized, or presented as separate facts/ideas without an overarching theme or argument from the beginning.

One consistent intervention that has been successful across multiple patients has been finding people (including therapists, peers, and parents) to whom they can verbalize their ideas. Possibly through doing this, patients can get help in determining salience through conversation with someone else. This can also help them to organize their own ideas by hearing them out loud and by debating out loud pros and cons of different structures and arguments. This can then lead to the successful structuring, synthesizing, and production of written work. Brett and Moira both still utilize this technique.

During this time, Brett learned that he loved to sing and excelled at it, could read slowly at grade level, but had excellent verbal reasoning and vocabulary. He still had low/average math skills, with no ability to see or read graphs/charts and therefore benefitted from math tutoring. Science was similarly difficult, and it was only through the use of external, accredited individualized classes that he was able to master the required material. *He was a very slow writer but had terrific innovative ideas. He continued to have trouble with executive function issues of planning and organizing, but was able to manage with the help of the school's learning specialist.*

When asked to reflect on her ongoing spatial issues, Moira endorsed challenges in *visuospatial awareness* (awareness of own body in space or personal space of others), saying "*If this includes having bruises you don't remember getting and bumping into things even in familiar places when you're not paying attention, that's me." Moira said she was very bad at drawing, or assembling objects, having to talk her way through requiring a great deal of effort and thinking really hard about visuospatial construction.* Visuospatial scanning and tracking, such as finding information on a page/poster/screen when there are a lot of distracting images or text, required a lot of training and talking to herself. Moira said she was not good at *spatial estimation* (judging distance, quantity, or time), appropriately using the space on a page. Her *three-dimensional thinking* such as route finding and following directions to a location is impacted. Moira had to learn (with a lot of work) how to *interpret information presented pictorially* such as diagrams, maps, figures, graphs, and analog clocks.

2.4 Considering Post-high School Options

Many children with NVLD will want to continue their education after high school. They will need help understanding how their disabilities might impact their experience in order to maximize success. A college counselor can help the family and student address important questions, what signs of trouble to watch for, and how to prepare. *Brett and his family met with a counselor who specializes in working with children with learning issues. She began the process of teaching Brett and his family the warning signs to look for and how to deal with his challenges himself. She asked them to consider if Brett was mature enough to move into a college dorm.* As many students with NVLD have difficulty reading nonverbal social cues, she wondered if he was aware of the level of his difficulty and if he had learned how to cope with the resulting confusion. Was Brett ready for the social give-and-take that is required to live with a roommate or would he be able to get a single room? *Brett requested a single room but then was given a roommate and had to have a lot of help dealing with the ensuing problems. She asked how well will Brett be able to handle exposure to sex, drugs, and alcohol. How would he know if he had a problem?*

Many students who have had social difficulties in the past are so eager to make friends that they are particularly vulnerable to peer pressure around drugs and alcohol. Similarly, they may be so eager to have a girlfriend or boyfriend that they place themselves in a situation where they can be taken advantage of. *The family was asked to consider if Brett was ready to take on the organizational responsibilities that are necessary when living away from home, such as managing money, doing laundry, eating healthy food, getting enough sleep, and getting to class on time. Systems were put into place to delineate the areas of mutual concern including learning and practicing the needed life skills prior to leaving home.* Professionals and parents should watch for and take action on these potential areas of concern.

A college counselor would be useful to guide the application process. Students with NVLD will need to understand the essential difference between the laws that govern K–12 education and the laws that govern postsecondary education which makes it the student's responsibility to self-identify and provide documentation of the disability (see McClure (2013) in "Treating NVLD in Children," Chap. 11, for more details). They will help to prepare for college admission tests (either the SAT or the ACT), or look into schools that are "test optional" (http://www.fairtest.org), and might benefit from a test preparation course or tutor.

Brett decided to only apply to schools that didn't require testing to reduce his stress. It is helpful to determine the level of accommodations and/or services the student will need and guide them through picking a college that will offer the best fit. *Structured* programs work best for students who need close monitoring and high levels of support. This is the greatest level of support provided on college campuses, and there are few institutions that offer it. Some of the hallmarks of this level are (a) staff trained to work with students with NVLD; (b) special orientation programs, usually before school starts; (c) some curriculum modifications offered, if this is supported by a student's documentation; (d) assistance with advocacy; (e) academic monitoring and counseling; and (f) professional subject area tutors rather than student tutors as they may be better equipped to help students with NVLD, given their special needs.

Coordinated services are the next level and work best for students who want to be "mainstreamed" but know they will need support. These services often include (a) instruction on learning strategies, (b) counseling/advising, (c) tutoring, and (d) assistance with advocacy. Colleges without any special programs offer only *basic* services. These programs provide the minimum support necessary in order to comply with the law (accommodations but not services). These colleges work best for the highly motivated, independent self-advocators. It is important for students with NVLD to know that it is the student's responsibility to self-identify and provide documentation of their disability. We need to help them become good self-advocates. *Both Brett and Moira decided to attend schools with only the most basic services, hoping for the best.*

2.5 College Years

Both Moira and Brett went on to 4-year colleges. Brett's choice allowed him more selectivity with the choice of classes with few requirements. He utilized all the tools he had acquired through his previous intensive tutoring and was able to succeed with only needing support for editing papers. Moira's college had many more required "breadth" classes. She found it difficult to pass the school's extensive science and math requirements. Seeking an explanation led her family to explore testing and treatment. Understanding her learning issues allowed her to work with her college to successfully make appropriate class substitutions.

Getting a late diagnosis, often however, results in the necessity of working through additional psychological issues created by the confusion and anxiety our patients often experience. *In Moira's case, she was initially suspicious, resentful, and very angry. Her family dynamics resulted in her experience that most of the family's resources for "help, attention, and therapeutic action" went toward a younger sibling, whose psychological issues required immediate attention. Moira had very strong feelings about this experience that she needed the space to express without judgment. Many hours were spent going over her history in detail, with new lenses to aid her understanding. Many confusing experiences were now able to be processed. She initially experienced relief as she had feared that she was crazy and was hopeful that now maybe something could be done to improve things.*

Moira regretted the late diagnosis: she lamented the lack of age-appropriate interventions and because she was already in college, there were a lot more immediate issues that she had to deal with pretty quickly, in terms of a fast-pace of academics, life skills, job hunting, etc. without years to build up skills and a team to help work on that. She believed that an early diagnosis would have allowed her to "keep my world more controlled and smaller and opened it up bit by bit. Whereas because I was diagnosed late, we actually had to fire-fight a lot with pretty high-stakes issues (compared to elementary school) and work on narrowing/controlling my world without a lot of support like living at home, etc."

Moira, frustrated by the lack of appropriate interventions, created a rubric for herself regarding how to successfully socialize, which included a variety of tactics. A key overarching theme to her rubric was to reduce the number of unknown/new factors required to successfully socialize, such as interacting mainly in 1:1 situations or in small groups, in quiet areas, preferably known ones. Relatedly, she specified that "if public transportation is required, use only 1 maximum new type of transport per new person interaction and built in and allow for clear margins for transport time" and additionally, "don't schedule any work that needs to be done before noon the next day, allow for sleep recovery."

Over time, Moira was able to express her disappointment and resentment directly with her family. Initially this was difficult and she had a hard time sorting through her complex emotions. She realized that the idea that she had something that she would have to deal with forever, as it wouldn't be cured and go away, made her very angry. Her family appreciated learning what they had missed and done wrong, and continue to try to be more helpful, and ask more specific questions about how they can help her. It is an ongoing, ever-improving process.

Brett and Moira are currently successfully pursuing advanced degrees in their chosen fields. While in graduate school, Moira found that a very low dose of an antidepressant that is a selective serotonin reuptake inhibitor (SSRI) helped her deal with the ensuing anxiety. Math remains problematic for both of them, with Moira saying she still can't add and subtract negative numbers and deal with decimals or fractions or a number line. Thankfully she has made life choices that mean she doesn't have to!

Both of them found that they were helped significantly when they were able to talk out loud their ideas. This technique helped in overcoming initiation issues and in synthesizing their ideas into a coherent narrative. They found that with complex writing, it was difficult to be able to figure out away how to really understand the arc of the narrative in a coherent clear enough fashion to be able to put it down without holes between the thoughts. For Moira, the use of a detailed outline and creating headings to break the task into smaller sections was very beneficial as well. She has also come up with a team of editors to help her make proper transition sentences. *Moira says she "comes up with my overall argument and main points for the whole thing at the beginning, into a bullet point list, and then from there I built a more detailed outline of each chapter and then write every chapter by working from that structure out."*

Brett, in Nonverbal Learning Disabilities in Children (Davis & Broitman, 2011*), says that he thinks that one's frame of mind has a great deal of influence on one's ability to overcome any obstacle. "To deal with my NVLD, I had to embrace the fact that* *life is a process. I had to learn that nothing is ever finished and that what I was ultimately working toward was the right to keep pursuing more. The reason why this is so important to realize is that a great deal of this 'process' can feel a lot like banging your head against a brick wall over and over again. To be good at it, you need to be able to relish small victories and have enough self-respect and confidence to know how to get back up and keep trying even when it feels impossible. Making breakthroughs in your personal struggle with NVLD is a lot like walking up a spiral staircase very slowly. It will feel like you are going around in circles, but what is actually happening is that you are re-visiting something from one level above where you were the last time the issue made itself known. Things feel repetitive and redundant, but ultimately small victories become large ones and you are doing things that you never thought possible."*

Research is mixed regarding whether students with NVLD are more at risk for psychiatric disorders, like depression, with some finding increased levels of depression (Brumback, 1985; Fletcher, 1985; Rourke, Young, & Leenaars, 1989) and others not finding that children with NVLD are at increased risk for psychiatric disorders (Forrest, 2004; Mokros, Poznanski, & Merrick, 1989). It is likely that these contradictory findings are due to methodological weaknesses in prior studies such as small sample sizes and unknown sample recruitment. The significant differences in age groups, race, and income among the different studies and differing definitions for diagnosis given the wide range of diagnostic criteria used in research on NVLD likely also contribute to the contradictory findings.

Regardless of prior studies, clinical experience has shown that with interventions, accommodations, and modifications, students with NVLD are often able to tap into their skill sets and experience success. As emphasized by Brooks (1991) and his concept of islands of competence, students with learning disabilities have relative strengths and weaknesses, and it is at least equally important that the student's strengths get recognized and enhanced as it is to remediate any relative weaknesses or deficits. For students with NVLD, skill sets might include acquisition of a second language, drama, certain aspects of the arts, language arts, and some of the language-based sciences. Generally the support team continues to be involved in the student's program if not via the Individual Educational Plan (IEP) process then sometimes utilizing the Section 504 laws. Transition planning becomes essential and decisions about further education need to be made. In our experience, students who have not become too demotivated, depressed, or demoralized from being misdiagnosed and misunderstood can move on to successful adulthood if they, with the help of their parents and coaches, choose wisely with special regard for their strengths.

Personal accounts written by people with NVLD suggest that adulthood may bring more successful interactions and relationships. Debbie Green, for example, in *Growing Up with NLD* (1999), writes of her joys as a teacher. Laurie E. Reed talks of her career as an occupational therapist in *Unaware: Living with Non-Verbal Learning Disabilities* (2001). These authors all emphasize that early accurate diagnosis and appropriate intervention is crucial to the well-being of the person with NVLD. In Table 2.1, samples of potential academic difficulties by domain and age, we offer an overview of the different potential challenges children with NVLD face in school.

Table 2.1 Samples of potential academic difficulties by domain and age

Grade	Reading	Writing
Prekindergarten	May not be able to recognize their own name	May not be able to write their own name
Kindergarten	May not be able to recognize letters or words	May not be able to legibly write letters or words
1–2	Trouble with reading decoding may have difficulty learning sound/symbol code, but do not have phonetic deficits	Handwriting is labored, slow, and difficult to decipher
3–5	Trouble with reading comprehension is identified when curriculum focuses on the main idea, author's tone, and interpreting idiom and metaphor	Complex ideas are unable to be translated into written work productions
6–8	Increased difficulty comprehension with saliency determination	Increased trouble organizing essays Trouble identifying supporting ideas in essays Trouble writing transition sentences in essays Trouble writing topic sentences Trouble following structure of an outline
9–12	Increased difficulty with reading speed and comprehension	Increased difficulty with transitions in essays and production requirements

Grade	Math	Science	History
Prekindergarten			*Area of strength*
Kindergarten	May have little number sense	Difficulty following spatially oriented scientific explanations	*Area of strength*
1–2	Trouble learning to tell time, value of coins, math concepts such as greater than or less than, and names of geometric shoes	Geographical understanding may be limited	*Area of strength*
3–5	Trouble learning procedures, fractions, greatest common factor, etc.	Difficulty reading graphs and charts	Trouble grasping cause and effect in order to explain timelines (in the presence of good rote memory for facts)
6–8	Difficulty understanding ratios, converting fractions to decimals, and calculating percentages	Difficulty writing interpretive section of lab reports	Difficulty with writing assignments
9–12	Difficulty understanding geometric concepts	Difficulty understanding concepts and reproducing procedures in chemistry and biology	Trouble organizing complex historical relationships Trouble identifying and supporting arguments and theories

Social Difficulties at Different Ages

Grade	Social
Prekindergarten	Separation anxiety may be more pronounced during transitions
Kindergarten	Might talk to themself and wander inappropriately Difficulty with circle time
1–2	Difficulty on playground Calls out Stands too close
4–5	Difficulty in cafeteria May be left out of invitations to self-forming social groups
6–8	Difficulty in groups Trouble understanding rapid social discourse
9–12	Transition to high school – new peers Hard to engage in back and forth conversation which becomes an integral part of adolescent social experience Trouble reading body language Burgeoning sexual interests that they are unable to manage in a socially appropriate manner – need explicit cueing about how much time they can spend looking at another person, etc. Social media experiences can be difficult for NVLDs to understand Interacting with pop culture requires social comprehension and integration of that social knowledge with language skills – the integration can be difficult for NVLDs Trouble internalizing social mores without explicit instruction Trouble understanding sarcasm which plays a larger role in adolescent social experiences

In Chap. 3, we present a research-driven model for NVLD with 11 potential subtypes. We then report on a proposed new name and definition for NVLD generated by a consortium led by Prudence W. Fisher, PhD, Division of Child and Adolescent Psychiatry, Columbia University College of Physicians and Surgeons.

References

Allen, K. (1998). *Star shaped pegs, square holes: Nonverbal learning disorders and the growing up years*. Livermore, CA: Good Enough Books.

Ayres, J. (1994). *Sensory Integration and the Child.* Western Psychological Services.

Brooks, R. (1991). *The self-esteem teacher*. Loveland, OH: Treehaus Communications.

Brumback, R. A. (1985). Wechsler performance IQ deficit in depression in children. *Perceptual and Motor Skills, 61*, 331–335. https://doi.org/10.2466/pms.1985.61.1.331.

Charles Schwab Website, www.schwablearning.org

College Admission Tests (either the SAT or the ACT)

Davis, J., & Broitman, J. (2011). *Nonverbal learning disabilities in children: Bridging the gap between science and practice*. New York: Springer.

Fletcher, J. M. (1985). External validation of learning disability typologies. In B. P. Rourke (Ed.), *Neuropsychology of learning disabilities: Essentials of subtype analysis* (pp. 187–211). New York: Guilford Press.

Forrest, B. (2004). The utility of math difficulties, internalized psychopathology, and visual spatial deficits to identify children with the nonverbal learning disability syndrome: Evidence for a visual-spatial disability. *Child Neuropsychology, 10*(2), 129–146. https://doi.org/10.1080/09297040490911131.

Green, D. (1999). *Growing up with NLD.* Albuquerque, NM: Silicon Heights.

Griffin, J., & Gresham, D. (2002). *Binocular anomalies: Diagnosis and vision therapy* (4th ed.). Oxford, UK: Butterworth-Heinemann.

Hale, J. B., & Fiorello, C. A. (2004). *School neuropsychology: A practitioner's handbook.* New York: Guilford Press.

Inhelder, B., & Piaget, J. (1964). *The early growth of logic in the child.* New York: W. W. Norton.

Johnson, D. J. (1987). Nonverbal learning disabilities. *Pediatric Annals, 16*(2), 133–141.

Levine, M. (2002). *Educational care.* Cambridge, MA: Educators Publishing Service.

Lipton, M. (2013). The physician's role in treating NVLD. In J. Broitman & J. Davis (Eds.), *Treating NVLD in children.* New York: Springer.

Martin, M. (2007). *Helping children with nonverbal learning disabilities to flourish.* London: Jessica Kingsley.

Mehrabian, A. (1971). *Silent Messages.* Belmont, CA: Wadsworth.

Mokros, H. B., Poznanski, E. O., & Merrick, W. A. (1989). Depression and learning disabilities in children: A test of an hypothesis. *Journal of Learning Disabilities, 22*, 230–244. https://doi.org/10.1177/002221948902200406.

Mooney, D., Newberry, S., & Kurtz, N. (2006). *Nonverbal learning disabilities: A guide to school success.* Wallingford, VT: Maple Leaf Center.

Palombo & Berenberg. (1999). Working with parents of children with nonverbal learning disabilities: A conceptual and intervention model. In J. A. Incorvaia, B. S. Mark-Goldstein, & D. Tessmer (Eds.), *Understanding, diagnosing, and treating AD/HD in children and adolescents: An integrated integrative approach* (Vol. 3, pp. 389–441). Northvale, NJ: Aronson Press.

Pam Tanguay's. www.NLDontheweb.org

Pennington, B. F. (1991). Right hemisphere learning disorders. In *Diagnosing learning disorders: A neuropsychological framework* (pp. 111–134). New York: The Guilford Press.

Piaget, J. (1972). *The psychology of intelligence.* Totowa, NJ: Littlefield Adams.

Reed, L. E. (2001). *Unaware: Living with non-verbal learning disabilities.* Self published.

Rourke, B. P. (1995). The NLD syndrome and the white matter model. In B. P. Rourke (Ed.), *Syndrome of nonverbal learning disabilities: Neurodevelopmental manifestations* (pp. 1–27). New York: Guilford Press.

Rourke, B. P., Young, G. C., & Leenaars, A. A. (1989). A childhood learning disability that predisposes those afflicted to adolescent and adult depression and suicide risk. *Journal of Learning Disabilities, 22*(3), 169–175.

Tanguay, P. B. (2001). *Nonverbal learning disabilities at home.* London: Jessica Kingsley.

Tanguay, P. B. (2002). *Nonverbal learning disabilities at school.* London: Jessica Kingsley.

Telzrow, C. F., & Bonar, A. M. (2002). Responding to students with nonverbal learning disabilities. *Teaching Exceptional Children, 34*, 8–13. https://doi.org/10.1177/004005990203400601.

Test optional colleges. http://www.fairtest.org

The NVLD project. https://nvld.org

Thompson, S. (1997). *The source for nonverbal learning disorders.* East Moline, IL: Linguisystems.

Volden, J. (2004). Nonverbal learning disability: A tutorial for speech-language pathologists. *American Journal of Speech-Language Pathology, 13*, 128–141. https://doi.org/10.1044/1058-0360(2004/014).

Whitney, R. V. (2000). *The nonverbal learning disorder guide for teachers, parents, employers, and therapists.* Campbell, CA: Lighthouse Project.

Chapter 3
What Is a Nonverbal Learning Disability (NVLD)

Our review of existing models of NVLD, along with our clinical experiences assessing and treating individuals with NVLD, led us to develop a neuropsychologically based model of NVLD that has 11 subtypes (Fig. 3.1). In our view, this improves on the four subtype model we presented previously (Davis & Broitman, 2011) because it allows for a more nuanced approach to characterizing potential subtypes and neuropsychological profiles of NVLD. In what follows we describe these profiles.

We consider visual–spatial deficits to be the primary components of NVLD, and they constitute the core deficits in the model. By core we mean that any child with NVLD would have these issues; in other words a visual–spatial deficit is a necessary, but not sufficient feature of NVLD. In addition to this single deficit, there must be impaired function in order to make a diagnosis of NVLD.

Based on prior clinical descriptions and research definitions, we think impairment occurs most often in four domains: motor development, executive functioning, math skills, and social skills. Most current research and clinical definitions of NVLD require that an individual has challenges in at least two of these areas along with the core deficit in visual–spatial processing (Banker et al., 2020; Fine, Musielak, & Semrud-Clikeman, 2014; Semrud-Clikeman & Fine, 2011; Semrud-Clikeman, Fine, Bledsoe, & Zhu, 2014).

Working within a model that visual–spatial deficits are the necessary, but not sufficient feature of NVLD, we hypothesize that there are 11 different possible variations of NVLD, formed by taking each possible combination:

- Visual–spatial and math/motor deficits
- Visual–spatial and math/executive function deficits
- Visual–spatial and math/social deficits
- Visual–spatial and motor/executive functions deficits
- Visual–spatial and motor/social deficits
- Visual–spatial and social deficits/executive functions deficits
- Visual–spatial and math/social/executive functions deficits
- Visual–spatial and math/motor/social deficits
- Visual–spatial and motor/math, and executive functions deficits
- Visual–spatial and motor/social/and executive functions deficit
  And lastly, children with all possible challenges
- Visual–spatial and motor/social/math/and executive function deficits

J. Broitman et al., *NVLD and Developmental Visual-Spatial Disorder in Children*, https://doi.org/10.1007/978-3-030-56108-6_3

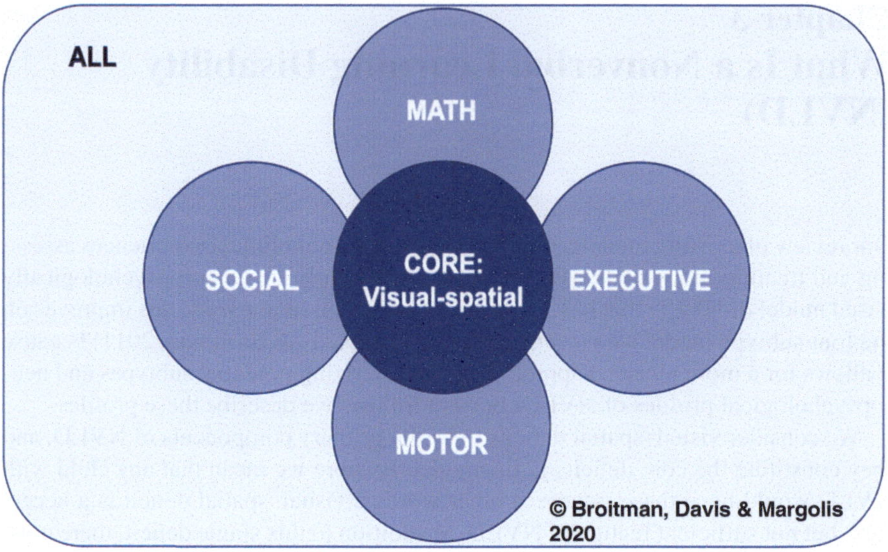

Fig. 3.1 Model of NVLD/Developmental visual–spatial disorder

We further theorize that certain profiles will present more prominently at different developmental stages and will be more commonly diagnosed at those ages. Some of these subtypes were described and illustrated by Brett and Moira in detail in Chap. 2, which covered the developmental signs of various NVLD models we describe below. In addition, we suggest a severity model in which children who present with deficits in all five areas will have the most functional impairment. These hypotheses warrant further investigation through rigorous research. We hope to address such questions in large datasets like the Healthy Brain Network (Alexander et al., 2017) wherein we can define individuals who meet criteria for NVLD and assess severity using independent measures of global functioning such as the Columbia Impairment Scale (Bird et al., 1993).

Using this research-based model for NVLD (Fig. 3.2), we recently completed a study of the prevalence of NVLD in North America. Until this study, there had not been an estimate of the frequency, or prevalence, of NVLD in a community sample. All prior studies examined the prevalence of NVLD only within samples of children already diagnosed with a learning disorder. These studies therefore might have grossly underestimated the prevalence of NVLD, since they were conducted within a restricted sample.

We conducted our study within three large samples of children who were enrolled in studies centered around brain imaging and the occurrence of psychiatric diagnoses or effects of maternal smoking during pregnancy. We applied our diagnostic criteria for NVLD to the existing test data for each participant in the study; we also adjusted the rates to match the census and correct for underrepresentation of individuals relative to the population. We also corrected for overrepresentation of

Table 1. Criteria for Nonverbal Learning Disability Diagnosis

Step, domain	Evidence[a]
1	
Visual-spatial deficit	Performance ≤16th percentile on visual-spatial tests or significant discrepanc between verbal and spatial abilities (eg, VIQ-PIQ ≥15 points)
Intact single-word reading abilities	Performance >16th percentile
2	
Social skills	Deficit in at least 2 of 4 areas: performance ≤16th percentile
Visual executive functioning	
Math calculation	
Motor skills	
3, Absence of ASD features	ASD features ruled out by survey or by study exclusion criteria

Fig. 3.2 Research criteria for NVLD
Measures used to determine eligibility for NVLD in three community samples (Margolis, Broitman, et al., 2020). *ASD* **autism spectrum disorder,** *VIQ* **verbal intelligence quotient,** *PIQ* **performance intelligence quotient. Originally published in Margolis et al. Estimated prevalence of nonverbal learning disability among North American children and adolescents.** *JAMA Network Open.* **2020;3(4)**

psychiatric disorders in the psychiatrically weighted samples by using a disorder inflation weight. Our findings suggest that 3–4% of children and adolescents in the general population meet the diagnostic criteria for NVLD. This translates to roughly 2–3 million children and adolescents in the United States who may have NVLD. Note that we excluded children with potential comorbid autism spectrum disorder in this study because we hoped to estimate the rate of NVLD separate from NVLD that might co-occur with ASD, as shown in Step 3 in Fig. 3.2.

Moreover, we also showed that the most common diagnosis that individuals who met criteria for NVLD received was ADHD, followed by anxiety disorder (Fig. 3.3). Additionally there was a subset of children in these studies who met criteria for NVLD but received no diagnosis in the comprehensive assessment conducted in the original study; such findings underscore the importance of NVLD being recognized as a distinct disorder to ensure that these children would receive a diagnosis and thus services and intervention.

Our findings that ADHD and anxiety disorders were most common in the sample who met criteria for NVLD are consistent with clinical anecdote and experience. It has been commonly noted that individuals with NVLD often have difficulty with inattention and executive functioning, as well as concern and worry about social and academic challenges, in addition to generalized anxiety and at times phobias or separation anxiety. NeuroBehavioral Institute, an outpatient and residential facility for obsessive compulsive disorder (OCD) and anxiety disorders in Weston, Florida, is well-known for its expertise in treating OCD. Through communication with one of the authors (Margolis), the NBI reports high numbers of individuals with NVLD seeking treatment for OCD. Interest in the disorder and its shared occurrence with NVLD prompted a joint workshop for professionals in winter 2019. We are currently developing ways to modify evidence-based treatment for OCD for individuals with NVLD, as described in Chap. 14.

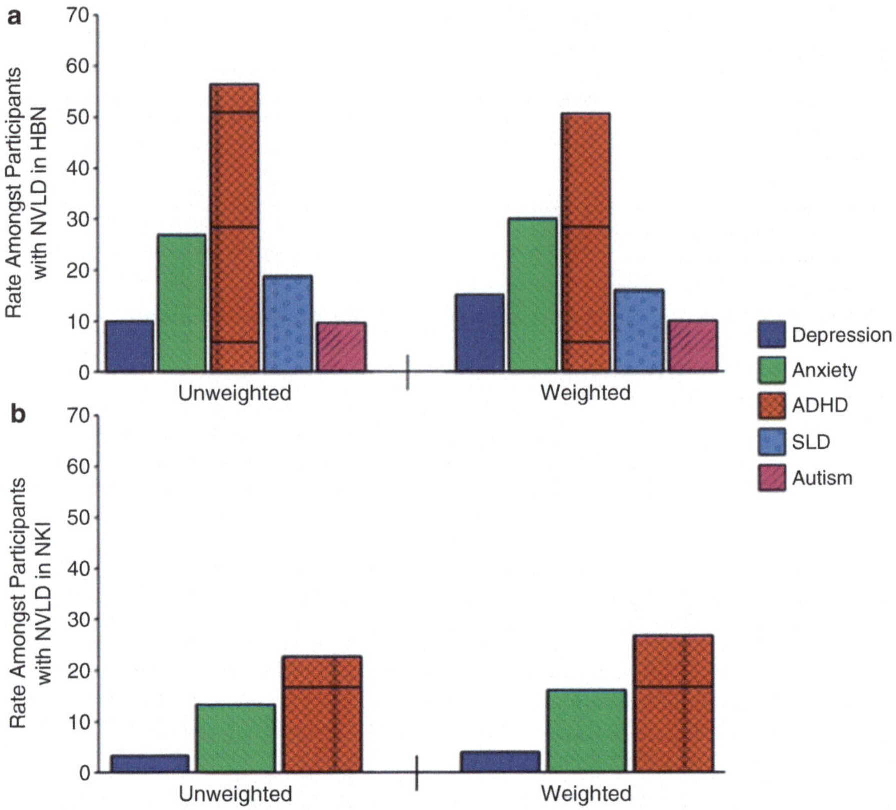

Fig. 3.3 Rates of disorders in NVLD
Unweighted and sample-weighted rates of psychiatric diagnoses among participants with nonverbal learning disorder in Healthy Brain Network (HBN) and Nathan Kline Institute (NKI) samples. Originally published in Margolis et al. Estimated prevalence of nonverbal learning disability among North American children and adolescents. *JAMA Network Open.* **2020;3(4)**

In addition to a research definition, the field has long needed a set of clinical criteria for making a diagnosis of NVLD. Until recently clinicians used their own judgment based on readings and case studies and clinical experience to defend a diagnosis of NVLD. Our 11 subtype model of NVLD that is based on research criteria is consistent with a new set of behavioral criteria developed through two consensus conferences held at Columbia University Irving Medical Center (CUIMC) in May 2017 and October 2018. This conference, sponsored by The NVLD Project, was led by Dr. Prudence Fisher and hosted at CUIMC. The consensus group included Dr. Amy Margolis, NVLD global experts, Drs. Jessica Broitman, Joseph Casey, John (Jack) M. Davis, Margaret Semrud-Clikeman, Jodene Fine, Irene Mammarella, and Doug Riis. The scientific advisors to the consortium include Drs. Michael Furst, Mark Riddle, Geraldine Dawson, Peter Satzmari, Stephen Hinshaw,

James McCracken, Benedetto Vitiello, and Agnes Whitaker. Educators from Mary McDowell School and Winston Preparatory School in NYC that offer programming for students with NVLD and policy makers from the National Center for Learning Disabilities (NCLD) also attended these meetings.

The central aims of the meetings were to generate a clinical definition of NVLD. To do so we defined a set of behavioral criteria for NVLD that could be submitted to the *Diagnostic and Statistical Manual 5* (DSM5) for consideration of NVLD as a distinct disorder. In addition, we identified specific empirical studies that would be needed before a submission could be made to *DSM5*.

Inclusion of NVLD in the *DSM5* could potentially improve a number of things for individuals with NVLD. Inclusion in DSM would provide improved identification of individuals with NVLD and thus communication among treating professionals. Inclusion would also provide access to care by allowing for billing for treatment. Currently individuals with NVLD tend to receive diagnoses that capture some of their functional impairments but do not signal the hallmark feature of NVLD, a visual–spatial deficit. *The International Statistical Classification of Diseases and Related Health Problems, Tenth Revision* (ICD-10) provides a code for individuals with visuospatial deficit (R41.842), which may capture NVLD. Last inclusion in *DSM5* would encourage and support research on treatment by having a clear set of diagnostic criteria.

Additionally, the conference focused on generating a name for NVLD that would be descriptive and would define NVLD based on its defining deficits rather than a description focusing on what it is not (nonverbal). The consensus group arrived at the name developmental visual–spatial disorder and generated a definition written within the style of *DSM5* diagnostic criteria. (See the appendices for a draft of the proposed definition.) In contrast to our research definition wherein criteria are defined by neuropsychological test profile, the clinical definition is based largely on behavioral features. Like several other neurodevelopmental disorders in *DSM5* (Language disorder, specific learning disorder, intellectual disability), NVLD does require some psychological testing to make a diagnosis.

The clinical definition is based on a single criterion outlined in the A criteria. The other B–D criteria specify that the deficits must have been present in the developmental period (although some may have been masked by superior overall intellectual abilities), cause specific distress and impairment, and are not accounted for by other conditions such as intellectual disability (intellectual developmental disorder) or uncorrected problems in visual acuity.

As defined by the consensus group, the A criteria for developmental visual–spatial disorder (NVLD) specify seven dimensions of visual–spatial processing in which an individual may have difficulties. In order to meet the criteria for the disorder, an individual must have problems in four of seven areas. One strength of the definition is the careful delineation of these seven aspects of visual–spatial processing. There are a few extant studies showing that relative to individuals with ASD or ADHD, children with NVLD have deficits in visual–spatial construction or processing (Mammarella, Cardillo, & Zoccante, 2019; Semrud-Clikeman, Walkowiak, Wilkinson, & Christopher, 2010). However, to date there is no comprehensive study looking systematically at low-level visual and higher-order visual–spatial processing in children with NVLD. The A criteria specified in the new definition provide a set of testable criteria.

The A criteria are described as persistent deficits in processing and integrating visual and spatial information. The criteria are to be met based on a clinical synthesis of the individual's history (developmental, medical, family, educational school reports) and psychoeducational or neuropsychological assessment. Moreover, for a diagnosis, the individual must have an impairment in some life activity in addition to meeting the A criteria. The following are the seven areas:

- Visuospatial awareness (e.g., awareness of own body in space or personal space of others, orienting to new environments)
- Visuospatial construction (e.g., copying visually presented material, planning, orienting, or organizing stimuli that are visual–spatial in nature, drawing, assembling objects))
- Visuospatial memory (e.g., remembering patterns and designs, recalling layout of environments, holding spatial information in mind while simultaneously acting on that information)
- Visuospatial scanning/tracking (e.g., finding information on a page/poster/screen, etc. when there are a lot of distracting images or text, locating things in presence of clutter, maneuvering in places or situations where other people or things are moving around quickly and in different directions)
- Spatial estimation (e.g., judging distance, quantity, or time, appropriately using the space on a page, allowing enough time to cross a street when traffic is coming)
- Three-dimensional thinking (e.g., imagining how things will look when rotated, route finding, following directions to a location)
- Interpreting information presented pictorially (e.g., diagrams, maps, figures, graphs, analog clocks)

By framing DVSD as a single deficit disorder, the consensus group sought to emphasize the importance of the visual–spatial deficit as the hallmark defining feature of the disorder. This also distinguishes DVSD from other neurodevelopmental disorders. Thus including DVSD will allow for millions of children to be identified as having a neurodevelopmental disorder that requires intervention. Currently, there are no diagnoses in *DSM5* that encompass visual–spatial deficits.

The theory of DVSD is that a deficit in visual–spatial processing lies upstream of the impairment, the associated difficulties, often detected in individuals with the disorder. This hypothesis is supported in part by evidence showing that in typically developing individuals visual–spatial skills are associated with motor, social, executive function, and math skills as well as symptoms of anxiety (Clements-Stephens, Vasiljevic, Murray, & Shelton, 2013; Frick & Möhring, 2016; Moriya, 2018; Mueller et al., 2009; Shelton, Clements-Stephens, Lam, Pak, & Murray, 2018; Young, Levine, & Mix, 2018), all areas that are impaired in NVLD. Further we have shown that the size of the verbal/visual–spatial discrepancy is associated with these outcomes in a large community sample of children (Margolis, Pao, Herbstman, Rauh, & Peterson, 2015). By showing that behaviors which are often impaired in individuals with NVLD are associated with a visual–spatial deficit, these studies support the premise that a visual–spatial deficit could be the core underlying feature of NVLD.

In addition to studying behavioral correlates of visual–spatial skills in typically developing individuals, studies have also examined these questions in individuals with NVLD. As described below, our research has documented links between dysfunction in the brain's spatial circuit and social functioning in children with NVLD (Banker et al., 2020). More research is needed to probe the behavioral and neural mechanisms underlying the link between spatial deficits and functional impairments that have been commonly reported in NVLD.

In Fig. 3.4, we hypothesize possible behavioral effects of spatial deficits on multiple other domains of function. The figure (©Margolis 2020) shows how a deficit in visual-spatial ability could underlie deficits in multiple domains. Notably, these problems in ancillary domains are often viewed as a primary deficit; thus, it is critical that we begin to understand the effects of visual-spatial processing problems on children's developmental trajectories.

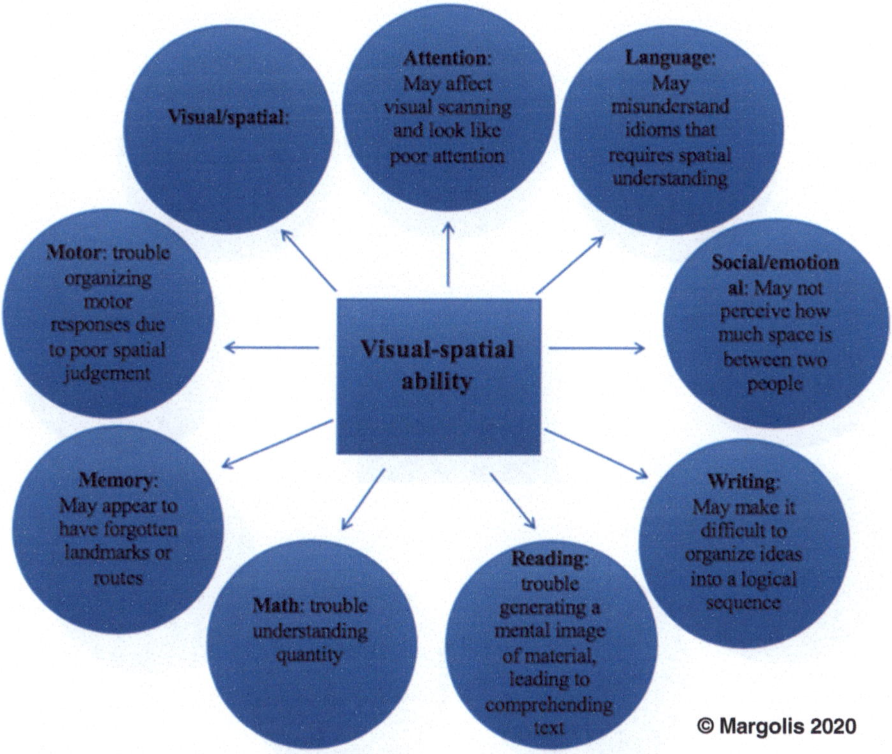

Fig. 3.4 A core deficit in visual–spatial ability may be interpreted as a deficit in a different cognitive, academic, or social function

The pathways through which visual–spatial deficits can lead to these other problems are not well understood. For example, problems in social function could derive from poor visual attention (does not see a raised eyebrow) or from conceptual interpretation (what does a raised eyebrow signal?). Similarly, if two people are standing close together, this could signal they are having a private conversation, but, if they are in a crowded venue, like a busy school hallway, this might not signal that privacy is being requested. Why does the child with NVLD have trouble understanding this? Does the child have trouble perceiving that the people are standing close together (perceptual deficit), or do they have trouble interpreting the meaning of the posture (conceptual deficit)? Future research must study these pathways in order to improve interventions.

Similar to how a deficit in visual–spatial processing can have downstream effects on other domains of function, in Figs. 3.5, 3.6, 3.7 and 3.8, we hypothesize how the impairments that are commonly associated with NVLD (problems with motor, math, social, or executive function skills) may affect other domains of function.

Figure 3.5 A deficit in motor skills may be interpreted as a deficit in a different cognitive, academic, or social function.

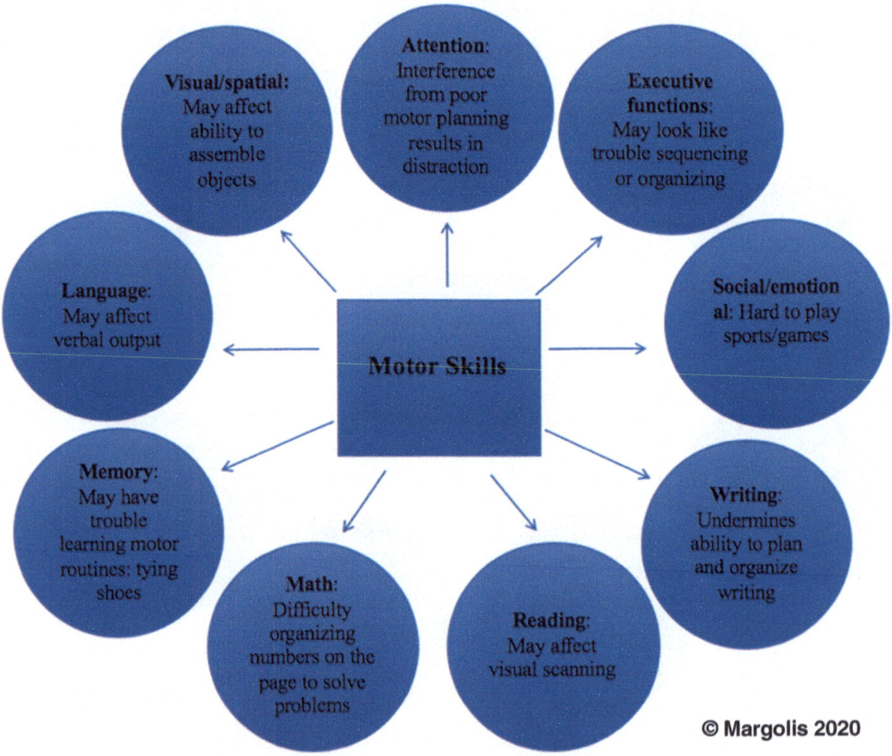
Attention: Interference from poor motor planning results in distraction
Visual/spatial: May affect ability to assemble objects
Executive functions: May look like trouble sequencing or organizing
Language: May affect verbal output
Motor Skills
Social/emotion al: Hard to play sports/games
Memory: May have trouble learning motor routines: tying shoes
Writing: Undermines ability to plan and organize writing
Math: Difficulty organizing numbers on the page to solve problems
Reading: May affect visual scanning
© Margolis 2020

Fig. 3.5 A deficit in motor skills

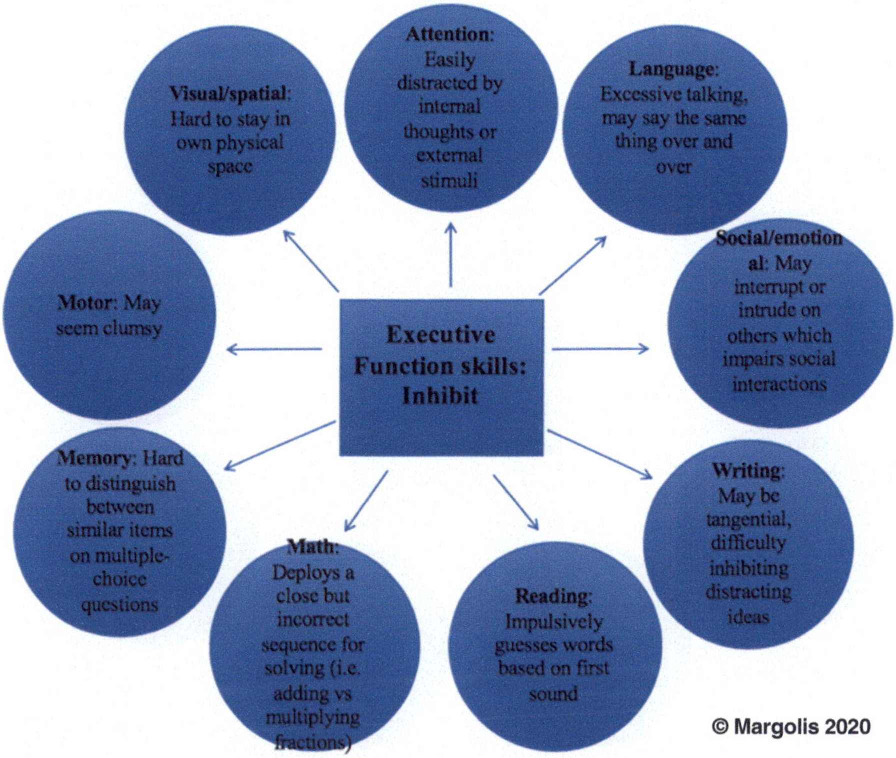

Fig. 3.6 A deficit in executive functions

Figure 3.6 A deficit in executive functions may be interpreted as a deficit in a different cognitive, academic, or social function.

Figure 3.7 A deficit in social–emotional function may be interpreted as a deficit in a different cognitive, academic, or social function.

Figure 3.8 A deficit in math skills may be interpreted as a deficit in a different cognitive, academic, or social function.

These figures show how important a complete assessment is in order to develop a comprehensive picture of an individual's strengths and weaknesses. A core deficit in one area (e.g., visual–spatial) may be overlooked or not recognized, and the assessment may instead focus on the more easily observed and commonly reported difficulties such as with social skills or math skills. In part we think this stems from the overarching lack of research and reports of visual–spatial problems in the literature. We often refer children to early intervention services for language delay during the toddler years, so too should we be referring for services when children have visual–spatial delays. This of course requires active research programs developing early intervention programs that can enhance visual–spatial skills.

Additionally Figs. 3.5–3.8 illustrate important ways for child neuropsychologists to conceptualize a profile of strengths and weaknesses. Reported difficulties in one

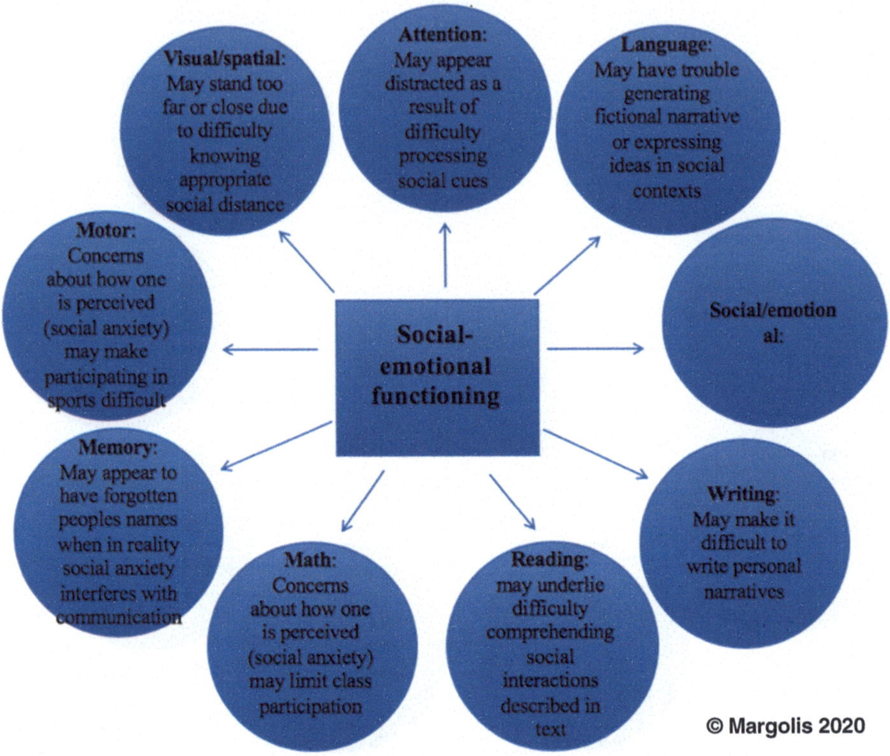

Fig. 3.7 A deficit in social–emotional function

area (e.g., attention) may actually reflect an upstream deficit in many different domains. Understanding the bidirectional nature of the interaction between deficits and outcomes is at the core of a comprehensive neuropsychological assessment and, thus, treatment plan. This approach is particularly important for NVLD which has a number of different presentations that we believe vary with the particular subtype of NVLD.

In the next chapter, we review what is known about the underlying brain basis of NVLD and consider etiologic factors that may contribute to the manifestation of NVLD.

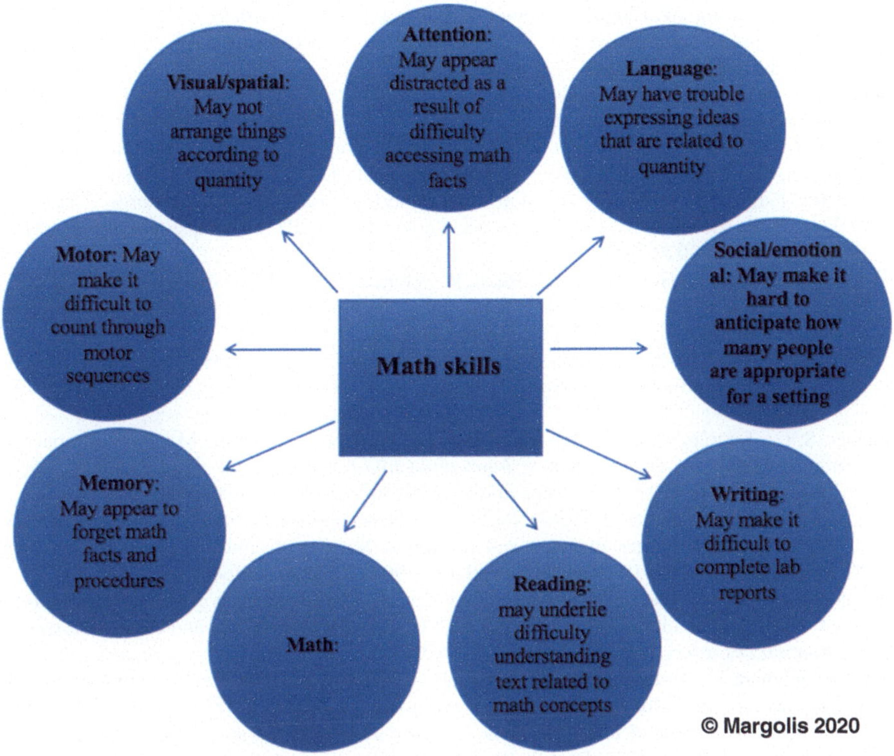
Attention: May appear distracted as a result of difficulty accessing math facts
Visual/spatial: May not arrange things according to quantity
Language: May have trouble expressing ideas that are related to quantity
Motor: May make it difficult to count through motor sequences
Math skills
Social/emotional: May make it hard to anticipate how many people are appropriate for a setting
Memory: May appear to forget math facts and procedures
Writing: May make it difficult to complete lab reports
Math:
Reading: may underlie difficulty understanding text related to math concepts
© Margolis 2020

Fig. 3.8 A deficit in math skills

References

Alexander, L. M., Escalera, J., Ai, L., Andreotti, C., Febre, K., Mangone, A., et al. (2017). An open resource for transdiagnostic research in pediatric mental health and learning disorders. *Scientific Data, 4*, 170181. https://doi.org/10.1038/sdata.2017.181.

Banker, S. M., Ramphal, B., Pagliaccio, D., Thomas, L., Rosen, E., Sigel, A. N., et al. (2020). Spatial network connectivity and spatial reasoning ability in children with nonverbal learning disability. *Scientific Reports, 10*(1), 561. https://doi.org/10.1038/s41598-019-56003-y.

Bird, H. R., Shaffer, D., Fisher, P., Gould, M. S., et al. (1993). The Columbia Impairment Scale (CIS): Pilot findings on a measure of global impairment for children and adolescents. *International Journal of Methods in Psychiatric Research, 3*(3), 167–176.

Clements-Stephens, A. M., Vasiljevic, K., Murray, A. J., & Shelton, A. L. (2013). The role of potential agents in making spatial perspective taking social. *Frontiers in Human Neuroscience, 7*, 497–497. https://doi.org/10.3389/fnhum.2013.00497.

Davis, J. M., & Broitman, J. (2011). *Nonverbal learning disability in children: Bridging the gap between science and practice*. New York: Springer.

Fine, J. G., Musielak, K. A., & Semrud-Clikeman, M. (2014). Smaller splenium in children with nonverbal learning disability compared to controls, high-functioning autism and ADHD. *Child Neuropsychology, 20*(6), 641–661. https://doi.org/10.1080/09297049.2013.854763.

Frick, A., & Möhring, W. (2016). A matter of balance: Motor control is related to Children's spatial and proportional reasoning skills. *Frontiers in Psychology, 6*, 2049–2049. https://doi.org/10.3389/fpsyg.2015.02049.

Mammarella, I. C., Cardillo, R., & Zoccante, L. (2019). Differences in visuospatial processing in individuals with nonverbal learning disability or autism spectrum disorder without intellectual disability. *Neuropsychology, 33*(1), 123–134. https://doi.org/10.1037/neu0000492.

Margolis, A. E., Broitman, J., Davis, J. M., Alexander, L., Hamilton, A., Liao, Z., et al. (2020). Estimated prevalence of nonverbal learning disability among north American children and adolescents. *JAMA Network Open, 3*(4), e202551. https://doi.org/10.1001/jamanetworkopen.2020.2551.

Margolis, A. E., Pao, L., Herbstman, J.R. Rauh, V., Peterson, B.S. (2015). Non verbal learning disability: Evidence for a discrete clinical entity in a community sample, 70th annual meeting of the Society for Biological Psychiatry. Toronto, Canada.

Moriya, J. (2018). Association between social anxiety and visual mental imagery of neutral scenes: The moderating role of effortful control. *Frontiers in Psychology, 8*, 2323. https://doi.org/10.3389/fpsyg.2017.02323.

Mueller, S. C., Temple, V., Cornwell, B., Grillon, C., Pine, D. S., & Ernst, M. (2009). Impaired spatial navigation in pediatric anxiety. *Journal of Child Psychology and Psychiatry, and Allied Disciplines, 50*(10), 1227–1234. https://doi.org/10.1111/j.1469-7610.2009.02112.x.

Semrud-Clikeman, M., & Fine, J. (2011). Presence of cysts on magnetic resonance images (MRIs) in children with Asperger disorder and nonverbal learning disabilities. *Journal of Child Neurology, 26*(4), 471–475. https://doi.org/10.1177/0883073810384264.

Semrud-Clikeman, M., Fine, J. G., Bledsoe, J., & Zhu, D. C. (2014). Regional volumetric differences based on structural MRI in children with two subtypes of ADHD and controls. *Journal of Attention Disorders*. https://doi.org/10.1177/1087054714559642.

Semrud-Clikeman, M., Walkowiak, J., Wilkinson, A., & Christopher, G. (2010). Neuropsychological differences among children with Asperger syndrome, nonverbal learning disabilities, attention deficit disorder, and controls. *Developmental Neuropsychology, 35*(5), 582–600. doi: 925868019 [pii]10.1080/87565641.2010.494747.

Shelton, A. L., Clements-Stephens, A. M., Lam, W. Y., Pak, D. M., & Murray, A. J. (2018). Should social savvy equal good spatial skills? The interaction of social skills with spatial perspective taking. *Journal of Experimental Psychology. General, 141*(2), 199–205. https://doi.org/10.1037/a0024617.

Young, C. J., Levine, S. C., & Mix, K. S. (2018). The connection between spatial and mathematical ability across development. *Frontiers in Psychology, 9*, 755–755. https://doi.org/10.3389/fpsyg.2018.00755.

Chapter 4
The Etiology and Pathophysiology of NVLD

4.1 The Etiology of NVLD

Many questions remain regarding the etiology of NVLD. What could be the underlying causes of NVLD? Genetic factors likely contribute to NVLD through their role in brain development and the formation of circuits that allow people to perform visual–spatial tasks and processes. Recent studies suggest that discrete aspects of intelligence, such as PIQ, are under genetic control (Guimaraes et al., 2020). There is also some evidence that the VIQ–PIQ discrepancy, which defines some patients with NVLD, may be under genetic control. In autism, verbal–spatial discrepancies are linked to two genes, one of which is also implicated in speech–language impairment (Chapman et al., 2011). In Prader–Willi syndrome, the presence of a verbal–spatial discrepancy depends on whether there is a deletion or uniparental disomy and is associated with higher risk for associated autism spectrum behaviors (Copet et al., 2010). The clinical anecdote suggests that children with NVLD may have ADHD, autism spectrum, or learning disabilities in their family history, pointing to a genetic risk for the disorders. Much more work is needed in this area.

Environmental factors, like exposures to neurotoxicants, may also contribute to the occurrence of NVLD. Recent studies document associations between prenatal exposures to neurotoxicants such as polybrominated diphenyl ethers or polychlorinated biphenyls (flame retardants), lead, or manganese and learning problems in general (Bhang et al., 2013; Cho et al., 2013; Cowell et al., 2018; Geier, Kern, & Geier, 2017; Margolis et al., 2020; Margolis et al., 2020; Miranda et al., 2007; Zhang et al., 2017). Components of air pollution (e.g., polycyclic aromatic hydrocarbons, PM 2.5) are linked with problems with attention and self-regulation (Cowell et al., 2018; Margolis et al., 2016), which are often present in learning disorders. Prenatal exposure to several components of air pollution including PM2.5 and black carbon has been linked with reductions in nonverbal (visual–spatial) intelligence (Chiu et al., 2016; Harris et al., 2015; Suglia, Gryparis, Wright,

J. Broitman et al., *NVLD and Developmental Visual-Spatial Disorder in Children*, https://doi.org/10.1007/978-3-030-56108-6_4

Schwartz, & Wright, 2007; Wang et al., 2017) suggesting a potential environmentally associated NVLD phenotype. In other words, environmental exposures may contribute to weaknesses in visual–spatial processing, which in turn may lead to the development of NVLD. Our ongoing research program is currently investigating how prenatal exposure to mixtures of common chemicals including air pollutants, flame retardants, and pesticides may be linked with changes in visual–spatial processing and potentially the occurrence of NVLD.

The pathophysiology, or brain basis, of NVLD is beginning to be elucidated. Several early MRI studies compared structural differences in children with NVLD to those with Asperger's and typically developing children. These studies produced findings suggesting a smaller splenium in children with NVLD relative to children with ADHD, Asperger's, and typically developing children (Fine, Musielak, & Semrud-Clikeman, 2014). In addition, children with Asperger's and NVLD had smaller anterior cingulate cortical volumes relative to typically developing controls (Semrud-Clikeman, Fine, Bledsoe, & Zhu, 2013). Lastly, children with NVLD had unsuspected cysts or lesions in the occipital region, whereas comparison children did not (Semrud-Clikeman & Fine, 2011). Further study is required to fully understand structural differences in the brains of individuals with NVLD and typically developing individuals.

The research program of the Environment, Brain, and Behavior Lab for Visual–Spatial Disorders, directed by one of the authors (Dr. Amy Margolis), aims to establish the pathophysiology, prevalence, etiology, and treatment of NVLD. We first examined structural and functional correlates of verbal–spatial discrepancies in typically developing adults and children, before beginning to study individuals with NVLD. With this approach, we hoped to understand how the brain supports visual–spatial processing in typical development before studying disordered processing. Once we had established typical processing, we could then try to understand how the brains of individuals with NVLD might differ from these typical patterns.

In a first set of studies, we examined brain structure and connectivity. First, we identified a brain network that appears to underlie the VIQ–PIQ discrepancy (Margolis et al., 2013). This network includes frontal and parietal cortices (inferior frontal, anterior cingulate, inferior parietal lobule, and supramarginal gyrus) that support cognitive control. Second, we found associations between verbal/visual–spatial discrepancy scores and a measure of structural connectivity in the brain (Margolis, Bansal, & Peterson, 2015). Specifically we detected positive associations between a measure of connectivity and the VIQ–PIQ discrepancy in tracts that could produce enhanced performance on verbal tasks and higher VIQ scores. We detected inverse associations between connectivity and the VIQ–PIQ discrepancy in tracts that could produce poorer performance on spatial tasks and lower PIQ scores. Thus, we detected patterns of structural variation in the brain that underlie verbal/visual–spatial discrepancies, supporting the idea that NVLD may also derive from changes in similar brain structures.

Last, using task fMRI, we studied how verbal/visual–spatial discrepancies might be linked with changes in how the brain *functions* during a visual–spatial executive function task. We showed that among typically developing children and adolescents, those with greater verbal relative to spatial abilities showed under-engagement of cognitive control regions that support executive function, specifically frontostriatal regions (Margolis et al., 2017). Our results suggest that individuals with greater verbal/visual–spatial discrepancies (as in NVLD) may have a combination of reduced conflict processing and difficulty selecting and attending to relevant stimuli. Such a pattern may also explain the behavioral and cognitive problems observed in NVLD; however we have not yet been able to explore this in children with NVLD.

In a second set of studies we acquired neuroimaging and neuropsychological test performance data from a group of children ages 7–16 years old who had a diagnosis of NVLD and from typically developing children. In these studies we have shown that children and adolescents with NVLD have reduced connectivity in brain networks that underlie spatial and social processing when compared to typically developing children, children with autism spectrum disorder, and children with reading disorder (Banker et al., 2020; Margolis, Pagliaccio, Thomas, Banker, & Marsh, 2019).

In the first study, we tested whether the shared social difficulties in NVLD and ASD might come from distinct underlying neurobiological pathways, in order to understand if the disorders have distinct brain bases. Specifically, we examined whether connectivity in the salience network, a brain circuit known to support social processes, differed between groups of children with NVLD and ASD and typically developing children. Our results suggest that the shared and easily observed social difficulties in the two disorders appear to derive from dysfunction in distinct parts of the salience network (Margolis et al., 2019). This work suggests that the two disorders are indeed distinct, at least at the neurobiological level.

In a second study, we examined the neurobiology underlying visual–spatial processing, the core deficit in NVLD. First we showed that a spatial circuit in the brain which has been validated in adults is also present in children. We then showed that the efficiency of the spatial circuit was associated with Performance IQ (PIQ) across the sample. Next we showed that both spatial processing (PIQ)) and global efficiency of the spatial network were positively associated with socioemotional functioning, supporting the hypothesis that deficits in spatial processing may underlie the social impairment observed in NVLD. Last we showed that relative to their typically developing peers and to children with reading disorder, children with NVLD have reduced functional connectivity within this spatial circuit (Banker et al., 2020). This last comparison to a clinical control group provides further evidence that dysfunction in the spatial circuit or brain regions that support spatial processing are specific to NVLD. Such findings point to a distinct neurobiological signature of NVLD, just as there is a distinct neurobiological signature of dyslexia (Chyl, Kossowski, Dębska, et al., 2019).

4.2 NVLD: Comorbidities

The proposed criteria for NVLD/DVSD follow the general principle of DSM5 that comorbidities often occur and that both diagnoses should be recognized and coded. The consensus conference group agreed that developmental visual–spatial disorder can be diagnosed in addition to the diagnosis of autism spectrum disorder, social (Pragmatic) communication disorder, attention deficit hyperactivity disorder, specific learning disorder, developmental coordination disorder, or any other mental disorder. Information for making a differential diagnosis (critical features that distinguish between two disorders) is also helpful for clearly describing a disorder. Next we discuss the features that NVLD/DVSD shares with other neurodevelopmental disorders (including autism spectrum disorders (ASDs), social anxiety disorder, attention deficit hyperactivity disorder (ADHD), and specific learning disorders (LDs), as well as how it differs from them. These features are also listed in Table 4.1.

The shared social difficulties in the ASD and NVLD likely underlie why their comorbidity has been of interest for many years. Children with ASDs and NVLD may share the following characteristics: dissatisfaction in social relationships, difficulty with reciprocal conversation, and difficulty identifying and interpreting facial expressions (Semrud-Clikeman, Fine, & Bledsoe, 2015). One older view was that Asperger's (now part of ASD) and NVLD were a single disorder that had been given different names by the psychiatric and neuropsychological disciplines, respectively (Kemp, Korkman, & Kirk, 2001; Klin, Volkmar, Sparrow, Cicchetti, & Rourke, 1995). However, as mentioned above, we recently showed that although parents' reported levels of social difficulties did not differ between children with ASD and NVLD, the brain dysfunction underlying such difficulties did differ between the groups (Margolis et al., 2019). These results point to different neurobiology underlying two distinct disorders.

In addition, there are some characteristics of ASD that children with NVLD do not have. Children with high-functioning autism (formerly Asperger's) demonstrate repetitive behaviors (hand flapping), fascination with parts of objects (spinning wheels, lining things up, collecting odd things), restricted interests, encyclopedic interests and knowledge of a topic (train routes, dinosaur names, features of the skyline), lack of spontaneous seeking to share enjoyment, interests, or achievements with other people (e.g., by a lack of showing, bringing, or pointing out objects of interest), lack of social or emotional reciprocity, and stereotyped and repetitive use of language or idiosyncratic language.

Children with NVLD and social anxiety disorder (SAD) may share concerns and worry about social interactions and social experiences. Characteristics that are specific to SAD and not NVLD include a typical neuropsychological profile, with good visual–spatial reasoning. Their academic profile is also not characterized by difficulty with math or science relative to reading and language-based academic tasks such as English and social studies class.

Children with NVLD and ADHD may both struggle in school with organization, academic demands, and dysgraphia. In contrast, ADHD is also characterized by features not shared across NVLD. Children with ADHD hyperactive/impulsive type will often have detectable hyperactivity and motor impersistence. Children with ADHD inattentive type tend to have an academic profile that is not characterized by difficulty with math and science relative to reading and language-based academic tasks such as English and social studies class. These children may miss details in class but can recount the gist. Children with NVLD tend to demonstrate the opposite pattern.

Table 4.1 Shared and distinct features of NVLD and other neurodevelopmental disorders

Disorder	Shared features	Divergent features (NVLDs do *not* have these difficulties)
All ASDs		
	Dissatisfaction in social relationships	
	Difficulty with reciprocal conversation	
	Difficulty identifying and interpreting facial expressions	
High-functioning autism/Asperger's		Repetitive behaviors (hand flapping), Fascination with parts of objects (spinning wheels, lining things up, collecting odd things), Restricted interests, Encyclopedic interest and knowledge of a topic (train routes, dinosaur names, features of the skyline)
		Lack of spontaneous seeking to share enjoyment, interests, or achievements with other people (e.g., by a lack of showing, bringing, or pointing out objects of interest), Lack of social or emotional reciprocity
		Stereotyped and repetitive use of language or idiosyncratic language
		Intact spatial abilities (no VIQ–PIQ split)
Autism		Language delay, in addition to behaviors listed above
Social anxiety disorder		
	Concern and worry about social interactions and social experiences	
		Normal neuropsychological functioning profile, such as good visual–spatial reasoning etc.
		Academic profile is not characterized by difficulty with math and science relative to reading and language-based academic tasks such as English and social studies class
AD/HD		
	Struggle in school with organization and academic demands	
	Poor handwriting	
Hyperactive/ impulsive type		Hyperactivity and motor impersistence

(continued)

Table 4.1 (continued)

Disorder	Shared features	Divergent features (NVLDs do *not* have these difficulties)
Inattentive type		Academic profile is not characterized by difficulty with math and science relative to reading and language-based academic tasks such as English and social studies class, miss details in class, but can recount the gist (NVLDs demonstrate opposite pattern)
Learning disorder in math (without comorbid reading or writing disorder)		
	Difficulty with concepts of numerosity	
	Difficulty with procedures for computations	
		Satisfying social experiences with peers
		Absence of social anxiety
		Good pragmatic language skills
		Good reading comprehension skills
		Good nonverbal communication

Children with NVLD and specific learning disorder in Math (SLD-M), without comorbid reading or writing disorder, may share difficulty with concepts of numerosity or procedures for calculations. In contrast, children with SLD-M likely do not have many of the features of NVLD including trouble attaining satisfying social experiences with peers, social anxiety, problems with pragmatic language, reading comprehension, or nonverbal communication.

Clearly, we have much more to understand in order to determine how best to intervene when helping individuals with NVLD and comorbidities. It is our hope that inclusion of DVSD in the DSM5 will lead to improved identification of individuals with NVLD and will encourage and support further research. In the next Chap. 5, we discuss the initial contact and intake process for diagnosing a student with NVLD. We outline the specific steps one must take to determine what treatment for a student with NVLD will need.

References

Banker, S. M., Ramphal, B., Pagliaccio, D., Thomas, L., Rosen, E., Sigel, A. N., et al. (2020). Spatial network connectivity and spatial reasoning ability in children with nonverbal learning disability. *Scientific Reports, 10*(1), 561. https://doi.org/10.1038/s41598-019-56003-y.

Bhang, S.-Y., Cho, S.-C., Kim, J.-W., Hong, Y.-C., Shin, M.-S., Yoo, H. J., et al. (2013). Relationship between blood manganese levels and children's attention, cognition, behavior, and academic performance—A nationwide cross-sectional study. *Environmental Research, 126*, 9–16. https://doi.org/10.1016/j.envres.2013.05.006.

Chapman, N. H., Estes, A., Munson, J., Bernier, R., Webb, S. J., Rothstein, J. H., Minshew, N. J., Dawson, G., Schellenberg, G. D., Wijsman, E. M. (2011). Genomescan for IQ discrepancy in autism: evidence for loci on chromosomes 10 and 16. *Hum Genet 129*, 59–70.

Chiu, Y.-H. M., Hsu, H.-H. L., Coull, B. A., Bellinger, D. C., Kloog, I., Schwartz, J., et al. (2016). Prenatal particulate air pollution and neurodevelopment in urban children: Examining sensitive windows and sex-specific associations. *Environment International, 87*, 56–65. https://doi.org/10.1016/j.envint.2015.11.010.

Cho, S. C., Hong, Y. C., Kim, J. W., Park, S., Park, M. H., Hur, J., et al. (2013). Association between urine cotinine levels, continuous performance test variables, and attention deficit hyperactivity disorder and learning disability symptoms in school-aged children. *Psychological Medicine, 43*(1), 209–219. https://doi.org/10.1017/S0033291712001109.

Chyl, K., Kossowski, B., Dębska, A., et al. (2019). Reading acquisition in children: Developmental processes and dyslexia-specific effects. *Journal of the American Academy of Child and Adolescent Psychiatry, 10*, 948–960.

Copet, P., Jauregi, J., Laurier, V., Ehlinger, V., Arnaud, C., Cobo, A. M., Molinas, C., Tauber, M., Thuilleaux, D. (2010). Cognitive profile in a large French cohort of adults with Prader-Willi syndrome: differences between genotypes. *J Intellect Disabil Res, 54*, 204–215.

Cowell, W. J., Margolis, A., Rauh, V. A., Sjodin, A., Jones, R., Wang, Y., et al. (2018). Associations between prenatal and childhood PBDE exposure and early adolescent visual, verbal and working memory. *Environment International, 118*, 9–16. https://doi.org/10.1016/j.envint.2018.05.004.

Fine, J. G., Musielak, K. A., & Semrud-Clikeman, M. (2014). Smaller splenium in children with nonverbal learning disability compared to controls, high-functioning autism and ADHD. *Child Neuropsychology, 20*(6), 641–661. https://doi.org/10.1080/09297049.2013.854763.

Geier, D. A., Kern, J. K., & Geier, M. R. (2017). Blood lead levels and learning disabilities: A cross-sectional study of the 2003–2004 National Health and Nutrition Examination Survey (NHANES). *International Journal of Environmental Research and Public Health, 14*(10). https://doi.org/10.3390/ijerph14101202.

Guimaraes, J., Bralten, J., Greven, C. U., Franke, B., Sprooten, E., & Beckmann, C. F. (2020). Discovering the shared biology of cognitive traits determined by genetic overlap. *NeuroImage, 208*, 116409.

Harris, M. H., Gold, D. R., Rifas-Shiman, S. L., Melly, S. J., Zanobetti, A., Coull, B. A., et al. (2015). Prenatal and childhood traffic-related pollution exposure and childhood cognition in the project viva cohort (Massachusetts, USA). *Environmental Health Perspectives, 123*(10), 1072–1078. https://doi.org/10.1289/ehp.1408803.

Kemp, S. L., Korkman, M., & Kirk, U. (2001). *Essentials of NEPSY assessment*. New York: Wiley.

Klin, A., Volkmar, F. R., Sparrow, S. S., Cicchetti, D. V., & Rourke, B. P. (1995). Validity and neuropsychological characterization of Asperger syndrome: Convergence with nonverbal learning disabilities syndrome. *Journal of Child Psychology and Psychiatry, and Allied Disciplines, 36*(7), 1127–1140. https://doi.org/10.1111/j.1469-7610.1995.tb01361.x.

Margolis, A. E., Banker, S., Pagliaccio, D., De Water, E., Curtin, P., Bonilla, A., et al. (2020). Functional connectivity of the reading network is associated with prenatal polybrominated diphenyl ether concentrations in a community sample of 5 year-old children: A preliminary study. *Environment International, 134*, 105212. https://doi.org/10.1016/j.envint.2019.105212.

Margolis, A. E., Bansal, R., Hao, X., Algermissen, M., Erickson, C., Klahr, K. W., et al. (2013). Using IQ discrepancy scores to examine the neural correlates of specific cognitive abilities. *Journal of Neuroscience, 33*(35), 14135–14145. 33/35/14135 [pii].

Margolis, A. E., Bansal, R., & Peterson, B. S. (2015, December 6–10). *Associations of White Matter Integrity and Discrepancies between Verbal and Performance IQ*. Paper presented at the 54th annual meeting of the American College of Neuropsychopharmacology, Hollywood, FL.

Margolis, A. E., Davis, K. S., Pao, L. S., Lewis, A., Yang, X., Tau, G., et al. (2017). Verbal-spatial IQ discrepancies impact brain activation associated with the resolution of cognitive conflict in children and adolescents. *Developmental Science*. https://doi.org/10.1111/desc.12550.

Margolis, A. E., Herbstman, J. B., Davis, K. S., Thomas, V. K., Tang, D., Wang, Y., et al. (2016). Longitudinal effects of prenatal exposure to air pollutants on self-regulatory capacities and social competence. *Journal of Child Psychology and Psychiatry, and Allied Disciplines, 57*(7), 851–860. https://doi.org/10.1111/jcpp.12548.

Margolis, A. E., Pagliaccio, D., Thomas, L., Banker, S., & Marsh, R. (2019). Salience network connectivity and social processing in children with nonverbal learning disability or autism spectrum disorder. *Neuropsychology, 33*(1), 135–143. https://doi.org/10.1037/neu0000494.

Miranda, M. L., Kim, D., Galeano, M. A., Paul, C. J., Hull, A. P., & Morgan, S. P. (2007). The relationship between early childhood blood lead levels and performance on end-of-grade tests. *Environmental Health Perspectives, 115*(8), 1242–1247. https://doi.org/10.1289/ehp.9994.

Semrud-Clikeman, M., Fine, J. (2011). Presence of cysts on magnetic resonance images (MRIs) in children with asperger disorder and nonverbal learning disabilities. *J Child Neurol, 26*(4):471–475.

Semrud-Clikeman, M., Fine, J. G., & Bledsoe, J. (2015). Social functioning using direct and indirect measures with children with High Functioning Autism, nonverbal learning disability, and typically developing children. *Child Neuropsychology, 22*, 1–18. https://doi.org/10.1080/09297049.2014.994487.

Semrud-Clikeman, M., Fine, J. G., Bledsoe, J., & Zhu, D. C. (2013). Magnetic resonance imaging volumetric findings in children with Asperger syndrome, nonverbal learning disability, or healthy controls. *Journal of Clinical and Experimental Neuropsychology, 35*(5), 540–550. https://doi.org/10.1080/13803395.2013.795528.

Suglia, S. F., Gryparis, A., Wright, R. O., Schwartz, J., & Wright, R. J. (2007). Association of black carbon with cognition among children in a prospective birth cohort study. *American Journal of Epidemiology, 167*(3), 280–286. https://doi.org/10.1093/aje/kwm308.

Wang, P., Tuvblad, C., Younan, D., Franklin, M., Lurmann, F., Wu, J., , et al. (2017). Socioeconomic disparities and sexual dimorphism in neurotoxic effects of ambient fine particles on youth IQ: A longitudinal analysis. PLoS One, 12(12), e0188731. doi:https://doi.org/10.1371/journal.pone.0188731.

Zhang, H., Yolton, K., Webster, G. M., Sjodin, A., Calafat, A. M., Dietrich, K. N., et al. (2017). Prenatal PBDE and PCB exposures and reading, cognition, and externalizing behavior in children. *Environmental Health Perspectives, 125*(4), 746–752. https://doi.org/10.1289/EHP478.

Chapter 5
The Initial Contact and the Intake Process

Referrals generally come from either a colleague, parent, school, or an individual who thinks or has been told they have NVLD. We do an initial consultation to determine the source of their concern. If relevant clinical data and neuropsychological testing exists, we request copies and read the material. If the testing is current and contains all the relevant information confirming a diagnosis of NVLD, we offer a consultation to review the current treatment in place to determine if it is meeting their needs. We would be looking for a pattern of results among the various tests administered to determine if any developmental or learning challenges emerge reflecting NVLD. Details on how to read a test report can be found in Chap. 6.

If there are insufficient test results to clarify the patient's strengths and weaknesses, we offer to gather more clinical information to clarify if testing seems warranted. This is done through an extended basic clinical interview that covers the patient's history of symptoms; medical, social, and school history; and all the normal psychological information we cover in an intake. The questions asked and rationale for the forms we use will be discussed below. The forms we use to gather the necessary data can be found in the appendices. If the data is suggestive of a NVLD syndrome (issues in visual–spatial; academic, math/science; social function; and executive function and environmental sensitivities), we would then make a referral for (or do) neuropsychological testing to confirm or disconfirm this diagnosis. Chapter 6, "Screening and Diagnostic Assessments for NVLD," delineates the specific tests administered. Once the results are available, one of us meets again with the family and patient to think through the next steps. If it is determined that the pattern of results is consistent with the diagnosis of NVLD, then we move forward to creating a treatment plan. If an alternative diagnosis is suggested, then an appropriate treatment plan or referral is made.

J. Broitman et al., *NVLD and Developmental Visual-Spatial Disorder in Children*, https://doi.org/10.1007/978-3-030-56108-6_5

5.1 Points to Cover in the First Session

We do a thorough intake using an ecological framework which includes first finding out what the primary concerns of the family are. What brought them to this place at this time? What worries, concerns, patterns of behavior, etc. are presenting as a concern? Then we take a family history, a developmental history, a social history, an educational history, and an environmental history, or what concerns/behaviors occurred in multiple contexts, and we try to obtain these from those who know and/or have worked with the potential patient, i.e., the legal guardians, typically the parents, relevant teachers, any therapists/speech pathologists/occupational therapists, and case manager(s) that might be involved. This could be done in a more or less structured fashion, but our approach is typically of the more structured variety.

There are a series of clinical questions that clinicians always need to ask and specific NVLD-related data that you will need in order to make your assessment. What follows are the specific points that we believe you need to cover in the first few consultation sessions. You will note that many of the clinical intake questions we utilize are similar to that of the intake for any neurotypical patient. In all treatments, one must develop an understanding of your patient's family dynamics and their psychology. Our typical consultation takes 2–3 sessions (reading reports and meeting with the family/patient) if current appropriate testing already exists. If not, then additional time will be required to allow for a 4–6-h test battery to be performed.

5.1.1 Reason for Referral

We will want to learn what led the patient/their family to seek therapy at this time. What are the patient's most pressing current problems? When did they first notice the onset and can they describe the course of the problem? How long has this issue (these issues) been going on? What is their understanding of the problem(s).

5.2 History

Try to find out about their and/or their families' current living situation, job, or jobs, health, and relationships with friends and significant others. Are the parents married or divorced, and do they have local family and other children? Learn about how their lives work. Gather a family medical history including current and past medications and psychiatric issues/hospitalizations and drug use/alcohol use. Has there ever been a psychiatric exam? What was their mental status? Were there any issues noted on the mental status exam? How was their affect? Any indication of depression or rage or suicidal ideation? What problems have the patient (or other family members) had in the past? If the patient has been in therapy before, what did previous therapists do that was helpful or harmful? Get a release to talk with their previous therapists.

Gather a family history including where they grew up and their socioeconomic status. Learn what you can do about the parents' personalities and the parents' relationship with each other. What is the parent's relationship with the patient like? What siblings are there and what is their relationship with the patient like? Explore their relationship with each parent and the nuclear family life, grandparents, cultural and ethnic issues, and religious issues, and ask for stories that talk about how it was to grow up and if there were/are any family traumas.

What is the patient's educational background? Where were they schooled from elementary to highest level? Were there any learning issues previously identified? Any notable school experiences and or issues or problems at school? Did they display expertise and/or have any passions or particular interests? Using your patients' passions and interests are the best way to help them move forward.

Have there been any physical Issues? Were all the normal developmental milestones met? Any health problems? How physically active was the patient? And what is their current physical involvement?

Are they sensitive to touch, light, taste, or smell or any environmental factors? In many cases, these issues can be "low hanging fruit" as there are low-cost, low-effort ways that sensory issues can be addressed. Therefore, it is important to check for sensory issues as part of a general diagnostic process for all of our patients.

At the end of an interview, ask yourself what you saw. Using your behavioral observations, how was your affect during the interview? Did it change at any point? What range of affect does the patient/family members exhibit? What were their affect cues and statements? How much of a crisis is the patient in? Is the patient suicidal? How worried do you feel about the patient? What is the patient's understanding of their current problems? How likeable is the patient? Can you emotionally connect or empathize with her/his problems?

Additional data we are seeking will come from the following checklists we ask the patient/family and relevant teachers to fill out. Copies for your use can be found in the appendices. Relevant forms are selected from the list below.

1. *The Children's Nonverbal Learning Disabilities Scale* (David B. Goldstein, PhD 1999) asks about motor skills, visual–spatial skills, and interpersonal skills.
2. *The Developmental Visual–Spatial Disorder* checklist addresses visuospatial awareness, visuospatial construction, visuospatial memory, visuospatial scanning/tracking, spatial estimation, three-dimensional thinking, and interpreting information presented pictorially.
3. *Scale of Executive Function* by Peggy Hock and Jane McClure © 2008.
4. Cornoldi, Venneri, Marconato, Molin, and Montinari (2003) *Shortened Visuospatial Questionnaire for Children* offers a glimpse of the child's own insight into their own difficulties.
5. Cornoldi et al. (2003) *Shortened Visuospatial Questionnaire for Teachers* captures the teachers' awareness of the presence of the NVLD symptoms in the classroom.

6. *Diagnosing Environmental Challenges* checklist helps us understand our patients' sensitivity to environmental factors that can cause daily stress. This can be very significant as small adjustments can make a huge difference to our patients' lives, comfort, and ability to learn and to function. Some factors are visible, while others cannot be seen. This checklist is also useful for breaking down/diagnosing how to best deal with a particular issue. Issues covered include sensory such as light, heat, sound, feel/touch, and taste. In the social area, there are the physical aspects, nonverbal aspects, logistical aspects, and psychological aspects to explore.
7. The *Sensory Modulation Scale* helps to understand if our patients have sensory sensitivities. It covers general modulation, over-responsiveness, under-responsiveness, sensory seeking, sensory discrimination, sensory-based motor abilities, social and emotional, and internal regulation.

While reviewing all of this information, we are looking for patterns or trends of what is already present and then figuring out what data might be missing in order for us to be able to render a reliable clinical opinion and/or diagnosis.

Next in Chap. 6, we address how to use neuropsychological testing to determine if an individual has NVLD. We describe the specific screening and assessment instruments we utilize and the areas we cover in our assessment battery.

References

Cornoldi, C., Venneri, A., Marconato, F., Molin, A., & Montinari, C. (2003). A rapid screening measure for the identification of visuospatial learning disability in schools. *Journal of Learning Disabilities, 36*(4), 299–306. https://doi.org/10.1177/00222194030360040201.

Goldstein, D. B. (1999). *Children's nonverbal learning disabilities scale. The children's nonverbal learning disabilities scale© was excerpted.* With permission from the author, from the Developmental Screening and Referral Inventory (DSRI) by David B. Goldstein, PhD, 1999.

Peggy Hock, P., & McClure, J. (2008). Scale of executive function. In J. Mcclure (Ed.) (2013), *College counseling with the NVLD student. Broitman, J, Davis, J.M. Treating NVLD in children: Professional collaborations for positive outcomes*. New York: Springer.

Chapter 6
Screening and Diagnostic Assessments for NVLD

In this chapter we will share our model for screening for NVLD and our model for a more comprehensive diagnostic assessment. Both begin with the traditional intake interview described earlier in the book. We then talk about our approach to screening, followed by what a comprehensive testing battery would look like, and end with the patterns of test data and how to share that information that may or may not support the existence of a client with NVLD.

While reviewing any preexisting assessments and parental information, we are looking for patterns or trends of what is already present. We then figure out what data might be missing in order for us to be able to render a reliable clinical opinion and/or diagnosis and/or deciding what more and what information might be needed. In certain circumstances (including limited resources), a family might want a less intensive exploration prior to committing to a full battery. In these circumstances we might first screen for NVLD. Our screening procedure follows the research protocols for identifying clients with NVLD (Margolis et al., 2020), which can then become a part of a more comprehensive battery if needed. The screening instruments we suggest are:

(a) A measure of intellectual potential, typically the Wechsler Abbreviated Scale of Intelligence-II (WASI-II) (Wechsler, 2011). This consists of 4 of the 10 subtests of the WISC-V (Wechsler, 2014) and/or the WAIS-IV (Wechsler, 2008) and takes about 1/3–1/2 the time to administer; the Full Scale IQ correlates in the low 0.90's for both of the more complete instruments.
(b) For academic testing we look for the WIAT-III (Wechsler, 2009) in large part because it is co-normed with the WASI-II. Here the basic reading or word reading and the math computation subtests are used.
(c) For the socio-emotional assessment, researchers have used both the Achenbach scales (Child Behavior Checklist, Teacher Report Form, and Youth Self-Report if 11 or older) Achenbach and Rescorla (2001) and the Behavior Assessment Scale for Children (BASC-3) (Reynolds & Kamphaus, 2015) rating scales

J. Broitman et al., *NVLD and Developmental Visual-Spatial Disorder in Children*, https://doi.org/10.1007/978-3-030-56108-6_6

which also has three different versions, one for a teacher, one for a parent, and one for the client to complete. These help to assess social–emotional difficulties as well as educational, attentional, and behavioral concerns.

(d) We also want to look more specifically at behaviors often associated with NVLD, so we use Cornoldi et al.'s Shortened Visuo-Spatial Questionnaire (SVS) Rating Scale (2003), a checklist for teachers aimed at collecting information about the presence of NVLD symptoms within the classroom environment. Since this is less well-known, we describe it in a bit more detail here. This questionnaire includes 18 items and uses a 4-point Likert scale (see Appendix 6.1). Ten items concern some of the deficits that, according to previous studies, represent critical features of NVLD. In particular, items include the child's use of the available space on paper while drawing; visuomotor coordination; comprehension of visuospatial relations from verbal description; coordination of complex movements; handling of the spatial components of calculation; orientation to space, drawing, visuospatial learning, and skills in observing the surrounding environment; and ability to deal with novel objects. These items are used to obtain a visuospatial score. The questionnaire also includes two items to evaluate aspects typically associated with NVLD, but these scores are not included in the total score. They concern handling of interpersonal skills (item 9) and mathematical learning (item 11). Two items (items 13 and 14) collect preliminary information evaluating the presence of comorbidity with ADHD (see Sandson, Bachna, & Morin, 2000). Finally, four more items are included as a control. They collect information on a child's verbal abilities (items 1 and 10), the teacher's estimate of the child's overall cognitive potential (item 17), and sociocultural level in general (item 18).

When conducting a comprehensive evaluation or supplementing a partial evaluation, we want to make sure that we are not only trying to diagnose NVLD but also addressing two other important areas. First is clearly stating whether or not the child/adolescent meets eligibility questions for Individuals with Disabilities Education Act (IDEA) to help parents to be able to request an Individual Education Plan (IEP) meeting with the public schools to try to get additional help for their child or for young adults to determine eligibility for the Americans with Disabilities Act (ADA) (see Chap. 7 for more detail). The Entitlement Law – IDEA (involves creation of IEP) – states that students with a disability are eligible for a free and appropriate public education if they need special education. The Individualized Education Program (IEP) is an individualized plan that establishes the educational goals for eligible students for one school year, created at a IEP meeting.

Below we offer a list of examples of ways we have linked visual-spatial deficits with functional challenges which can be helpful when arguing for services or accommodations. In it, we clarify the impact of visual-spatial deficits on an individual's functioning at home, in class, with peers, and in the community. Visual-spatial deficits (quantified by standardized tests of cognitive ability) can pervade all aspects of an individual's daily life and significantly impact daily functioning.

(1) Visual-spatial deficits can underlie problems with locational directions, maps, and orienting oneself in space. Having to travel to a new place or to a familiar

place independently can be very challenging, resulting in extreme anxiety. These individuals need to prepare multiple sets of plans (with parents or other supporting people) beforehand. When walking from their home, traveling on the subway or metro, or taking a city bus, they cannot look at a map or interpret directions independently to get from place to place.

(2) Visual-perceptual deficits affect all academic domains.
   (a) When reading, these deficits mean it is very hard to visually discriminate between the lines they are reading and the lines that need to be filtered out as they work on comprehending the broader text. They can also have trouble visualizing what they reads in their mind's eye, thereby affecting comprehension. They need to effortfully engage strategies for visual attention and discrimination in order to take in all of the information on the page, and having to engage those strategies takes time. When taking notes on reading, they have a hard time visualizing an outline or other appropriate structure for notes on the page. Individuals must use strategies to visually organize notes to make them useable and understandable. Putting those strategies into place adds time to each assignment.
   (b) When working on math, they often become overwhelmed by the amount of visual details on a page and cannot get started on calculations without engaging purposeful strategies. They need time to cover up all of the problems but the one they are working on (e.g., covering the page with a plain piece of paper or a folder) and then assign verbal labels to each part of the problem so that they can process and understand what is being asked. They require strategies to mitigate the effects of their visual-spatial deficits on academic learning, but implementing those strategies is time consuming and requires them to spend more time completing tasks than their peers.

(3) Visual-spatial deficits can make it hard for individuals with NVLD to organize material. Organization has an inherent spatial demand as sequences and relationships between items or ideas must be considered or made clear in writing, etc. Individuals with NVLD often spend a lot of time trying to organize activities and ideas, and that time is not always completely productive. They sometimes fixate on how their deficits will make a task hard and then can become overwhelmed by thinking about how to manage the task or set of tasks, all of which require organization and visual-spatial processing. They can attempt to use strategies to organize materials, ideas, and approach to tasks so that they can get started. All of this means that they spend more times on these executive functions than do typically developing age peers.

(4) Individuals with NVLD often become anxious when faced with novelty and when trying to process visual-spatial information. Before they can get started on things (making a homework plan, working on an assignment, discussing a confusing interaction with a teacher, clarifying task instructions, processing, and problem-solving unsuccessful peer interactions), they need to express worries about things that felt outside of their control. Without a plan in place, they have trouble envisioning themselves successfully completing a task, initiating a successful conversation, or coming up with a solution to a problem mid-task. They need strategies for regulating anxiety, balancing the demands of situations that are inside and outside of one's control, and developing sets of strategies

that they can use in different types of situations to structure the approach, get started without the help of an adult or peer, and navigate novel, uncertain information or instructions. Using these strategies is not automatic for individuals with NVLD, and thus they need time to effortfully put activate strategies.

(5) Visual-spatial deficits can also affect one's social life, peer interactions, and interactions with teachers. When faced with spatial challenges or with novelty (e.g., purely visual or spatial tasks, activities with which they are unfamiliar) individuals with NVLD can have a hard time controlling their worry, and that worry leads to other symptoms including frustration, difficulty concentrating, and difficulty shifting or becoming "stuck." Deficits in visual attention and spatial reasoning can interfere with social communication and ability to read nonverbal cues. For example, individuals with NVLD can have a tendency to talk continuously rather than leaving space for others to respond to what they are saying or to participate in back and forth conversations. They also can get "stuck" on one topic of conversation and have difficulty shifting to new topics. These difficulties, stemming from significant difficulties such as reading visual cues and recruiting their executive functions (shifting/mental flexibility), prevent them from connecting with classmates, asking for help from peers when struggling with a concept or a problem, and limiting ability to learn from peer models. Notably, most individuals with NVLD are aware of these social difficulties and feel anxious in many social situations, both academic and nonacademic. Such anxiety makes it hard to approach peers in the school hallway, initiate conversations, and listen to and process what their peers are saying when they do successfully enter into conversations.

And second, we believe that a comprehensive test battery needs to be able to answer other clinically relevant questions such as what are this particular student's strengths and challenges; what do the patterns of the results suggest in terms of interventions and/or accommodations; and, perhaps most importantly, how do we best *understand* this student so that we can help educate the parent and child to become their own best advocates. In order to do this, we use and recommend the following tests, although other similar tests can be used.

In other writings (Broitman & Davis, 2013), we have listed what we believe are essential areas to be assessed to complete a comprehensive evaluation. We include an updated version of that here in Table 6.1, followed by a list of the possible tests we use to measure these areas.

To assess NVLD we evaluate test data by looking for a particular pattern of results. We propose that it is extremely important to think in terms of case specificity while trying to synthesize the information gathered during the evaluation of clients with NVLD. The job of the clinician is to formulate case thinking about all the possible combinations of factors in a person's life. Pattern analysis is essential in understanding and then diagnosing an individual. There are strengths and compensating strategies that need to be recognized while focusing on recommendations for interventions and support. In summary the areas that are key to the comprehensive assessment, diagnosis, and understanding of NVLD clients are:

(a) Visual spatial intellectual abilities inferior to the normative sample or one's own verbal reasoning abilities, e.g., visual spatial intelligence (WISC-V: VSI) less

Table 6.1 Broitman, Davis & Margolis assessment battery (2020)

Academic testing: Math	
	Math concepts
	Math calculation
	Math application
	Math fluency
Academic testing: Written expression	
	Handwriting fluency
	Spelling
	Compositional fluency
	Writing mechanics
	Composition:
	Narrative and expository
Academic testing: Reading	
	Reading comprehension: Both literal and inferential
	Word identification or basic reading skills
	Fluency
Intellectual abilities	
	Verbal or crystalized
	Fluid/pattern analysis
	Visuospatial
	Quantitative
Language – receptive	
	Phonemic
	Awareness
	Morphological
	Syntax
	Semantics
	Pragmatics
	Receptive vocabulary
Language – expressive	
	Rapid naming
	Expressive vocabulary
	Pragmatics
	Verbal fluency
Memory – visual	
	Concrete vs. abstract
	Recognition vs. retrieval
	Sequential vs. non-sequential
	Immediate vs. working vs. long term
Memory – verbal	
	Contextual vs. de-contextual
	Recognition vs. retrieval

(continued)

Table 6.1 (continued)

	Sequential vs. non-sequential
	Immediate vs. working vs. long term
Executive functions	
	Cognitive flexibility
	Initiation
	Working memory
	Planning/organizing
	Internalized
	Externalized
	Self-monitoring
	Task completion
	Sequencing
	Switch between sets of information
Attention	
	Attention/focus
	Concentrate
	Sustain attention
	Maintain and direct optimal arousal
	Select information to attend
	Visual scanning
Sensory motor	
	Bilateral
	Efficiency
	Simple vs. complex
	Timed vs. untimed
	Sequential vs. non-sequential
	Proprioceptive
	Pencil grip
Sensory processing	
Sensitivities such as light, heat, tactile	
	Sensory profile
Visual processing	
	Sequential vs. non-sequential
	Timed vs. untimed
	Orthographic processing
Graphomotor – Timed	
	Grapho – symbol
	Grapho – non-symbol
	Handwriting
Graphomotor – untimed	
	Design
	Drawing
	Handwriting

(continued)

Table 6.1 (continued)

Affect and behavior	
	Depression
	Anxiety
	Thought problems
	Social problems
	Attention problems
	Oppositional behaviors
	Conduct disorder
	Self-esteem

than the 16th percentile or VSI less than verbal comprehension and reasoning (WISC-V: VCI) by 15 or more standard points.

(b) Basic word reading skills greater than the 16th percentile (WAIT-III: Word Reading).

(c) Social skill deficits on behavioral or adaptive rating scales at greater than the 84th percentile (Achenbach, BASC-III, ABAS- 3, etc.).

(d) Visual executive function deficits defined as scores less than the 16th percentile or a statistically significant discrepancy between visual and verbal scores (D-KEFS, design fluency vs. verbal fluency, and/or RCFT vs. CVLT, and/or WRAML-2, finger windows vs. number letter, and/or WNV, spatial span vs. WISC-V, digit span, etc.)

(e) Math calculation with score less than the 16th percentile or a significant discrepancy with math calculation a standard deviation below basic word reading (WIAT-III: math calculation vs. basic word reading).

(f) Visual motor skill deficits with results less than the 16th percentile (RCFT, VMI-6, etc.) or other supporting data from history or evaluations from physical therapists or occupational therapists.

(g) It is also important to consider impairment in associated areas that have anecdotal/clinical support for being part of the downstream effects of NVLD on an individual. Thus we recommend also including measures or questions/assessment of environmental factors/sensory processing, pragmatic language, understanding the big picture, handling novelty, and tactile perception.

(Note: A child does not need to have deficits in all of the above areas in order to meet criteria for NVLD and typically won't.)

Below we present specific tests that can be used to address the areas needed to assess NVLD. Within each area there are multiple measures listed because there are often more than one option to assess a particular construct or because different measures are available for different age groups. Selecting appropriate measures requires clinical judgment, and it is beyond the scope of this text to explain the process of selecting measures based on psychometric properties, etc.

Nevertheless, in Table 6.2, we list measures used in our sample assessment that would include a combination of the following tests that cover each of the domains listed in the table above in order to fully assess for the presence of NVLD.

Table 6.2 Tests that cover each of the domains to assess for the presence of NVLD

1. Academic testing:
a. Wechsler Individual Achievement Tests-III I (Wechsler, 2009)
This has subtests that measure listening comprehension, oral expression, basic word reading, reading comprehension, reading fluency, pseudoword reading, spelling, written expression, numerical operations, math reasoning, and math fluency
b. Gray Oral Reading Test-5 (6–23 years) (Wiederholt & Bryant, 2012) Rate, Accuracy, Comprehension
c. Nelson Denny Reading Test- 2 (high school to 4-year college) (Brown, Fishco, & Hanna, 1993) Vocabulary, Rate, Comprehension
d. Test of Word Reading Efficiency-II (Torgesen et al., 2012): Word and Nonword reading speed
e. The Berninger Writing Fluency (Berninger, 2007) a task for a quick measure of writing fluency
f. The Feifer Assessment of Math (Feifer & Clark, 2018): This relatively new battery has a variety of measures associated with both the academics of math and what is believed to be many of the underlying processes associated with math. We believe that it is likely to become more available and more used when testing students with NVLD and math deficits
g. KeyMath -3 (Connolly, 2007)
This assessment also measures essential math concepts and skills required for successful mathematical achievement
2. Intellectual testing (measures thinking skills)
a. Wechsler Intelligence Scale for Children-V (WISC-V) (Wechsler, 2014)
b. Wechsler Adult Intelligence Scale-IV (WAIS-IV) (Wechsler, 2008)
c. Wechsler Abbreviated Scale of Intelligence-II (WASI-II) (Wechsler, 2011)
These tests measure verbal comprehension or reasoning, spatial reasoning, visual/graphomotor processing efficiency, fluid reasoning, quantitative reasoning, and short-term and working memory. Each includes a different number of subtests to generate a Full Scale IQ score, and each has different index scores with different names. Particularly relevant to making a diagnosis of NVLD is the distinction between Performance IQ (WASI), PRI (Perceptual Reasoning Index on the WISC-V and WAIS-IV), and the Fluid Reasoning Index (WISC-V)
d. Differential Ability Scales-II (Elliot, 2007)
This is another measure of intellectual reasoning for children and adolescence. In the states under the Federal 9th Circuit Court where the Larry P decision negated the use of intellectual reasoning measures for African American students in the public school, this test is often allowed to be used as it was published after the ruling. It measures verbal, spatial, and fluid reasoning as well as some processing measures
3. Measures of Language Processing
a. Clinical Evaluation of Language Functioning-5 (Wiig, Semel, and Secord (2013)
The CELF-5 assesses the fundamentals of language like expressive, receptive, semantic, etc., utilizing nine different subtests. What this fifth edition also provides is another four subtests measuring the metalinguistic tasks often key to understanding the pragmatic issues accompanying some students with NVLD. In particular this evaluates making inferences, conversation skills, multiple meanings, and figurative language
b. Comprehensive Assessment of Spoken Language-2 (Carrow-Woolfolk, 2017)
The CASL-2 also assesses a broad base of language functions (14 subtests) and also looks into those pragmatic areas of idiomatic language, nonliteral language, inference, double meaning, and pragmatic language

(continued)

Table 6.2 (continued)

c. Test of Pragmatic Language-2 (Phelps-Terasaki & Phelps-Gunn, 1992)
Unlike the other tests just mentioned, the TOPL-2 is standardized for only one overall score. However, it does provide different item numbers which "tap" a variety of pragmatic issues which they claim can be used for intra-individual interpretation and strengths and weaknesses
4. Measures of cognitive processing
a. NEPSY-II (Korkman, Kirk, & Kemp, 2007) – a neuropsychological test for children 3–16 to access executive functions, language processing, sensorimotor skills, visuospatial skills, and a variety of memory abilities
b. Wide Range Assessment of Memory and Learning-2nd edition (Sheslow & Adams, 2003)
This test measures a number of aspects of memory with the traditional visual and verbal memory tasks and also looks at immediate recall, delayed recall, and recognition recall. There are comparisons available that are useful in the diagnosis of NVLD, particularly comparing the Design Memory and Verbal Learning subtest results and the Finger Windows and Number Letter subtest results
c. California Verbal Learning Test – Children's Version or Adult Version (Delis, Kramer, Kaplan, & Ober, 1994)
This is a verbal learning list task very similar to the WRAML-2 Verbal Learning subtest but has more options in terms of clinical scores that can be useful
d. Rey Complex Figure Test (Meyers & Meyers, 1995)
This is a complex design memory task often used in conjunction with the CVLT. The Rey is often given to students suspected of having NVLD. In particular, the Rey has been one of the more popular tests used in the research on NVLD, and having the contrasting verbal and visual tasks is always something we look at to further clarify and solidify a diagnosis of NVLD
e. Wide Range Assessment of Visual Motor Abilities (Adams & Sheslow, 1995)
This battery of tasks tests spatial, motor, and visual motor processing skills
f. The Beery Visual–Motor Integration Test-6th edition (Beery & Beery, 2010)
This is one of the more popular of visual motor integration measures and now also has motor and visual subtests available to try to parse out those issues if a student does poorly on the integration task
g. Delis–Kaplan Executive Function System (Delis, Kaplan, & Kramer, 2001)
This battery tests a range of executive function skills such and is currently the most comprehensive battery for these skills
h. Spatial Span
This is a visual working memory test found in the Wechsler Nonverbal Scale of Ability (Wechsler & Naglieri, 2006) among other places. Like the Rey Complex Figure Test, Spatial Span is one of the more commonly used tests found in the research on NVLD and is often compared with the Wechsler Digit Span tests to look for the "typical" pattern of students with NVLD of verbal task performance being superior to visual spatial tasks
i. Conners' Continuous Performance Test III (Conners, 2014)
This computerized task takes measures of attention, impulsivity, sustained attention, and vigilance
j. Developmental Eye Movement Test (Richman & Garzia, 2015)
This is a screening test typically used by developmental optometrists to check for tracking problems (up to 8th grade) among children
k. Comprehensive Test of Phonological Processing-2 Wagner, Torgesen, Rashotte, & Pearson, 2013): This battery tests for the processing areas of phonological awareness, phonological memory, and rapid naming, typically areas of relative strengths for students with NVLD

(continued)

Table 6.2 (continued)

5. A standardized measure of sensory processing
a. Sensory Profile 2 (Dunn, 2014)
In the previous chapter, a number of questions focused on areas of sensitivity of sensory processing which may be impacting our NVLD clients. The Sensory Profile™ 2 is a family of assessments providing *standardized* tools to help evaluate a child's sensory processing patterns in the context of home-, school-, and community-based activities
6. Measures of socio-emotional and behavioral functioning
a. Achenbach Child Behavior Checklist (Achenbach & Rescorla, 2001). The Achenbach series consists of three scales focusing on a wide range of behaviors, attitudes, and feelings:
Parent (Child Behavior Rating Scale)
Teacher (Teacher Report Form)
Self-report (Youth Self-Report)
b. Behavior Assessment Scale for Children (BASC-3) (Reynolds & Kamphaus, 2015)
The BASC series also has three scales, again the parent, teacher, and self-scales, and also focuses on a wide range of behaviors, attitudes, and feelings
c. Conners' Rating Scales (Conners, 2008)
The Conners' series also has three scales, again the parent, teacher, and self-scales, and also focuses on a wide range of behaviors, attitudes, and feelings
d. Behavior Rating Inventory of Executive Functioning-2 (BRIEF-2) (Gioia, Isquith, Guy, & Kenworthy, 2015)
The BRIEF-2 is a more specialized scale focusing on a variety of what the research generally refers to as executive functioning
e. Vineland Adaptive Behavior Scales-3 (Sparrow, Cicchetti, & Saulnier, 2016)
This rating scale is devoted to measuring aspects of adaptive functioning in the areas of communication, daily living skills, and motor skills and is administered to parents and teachers
f. Adaptive Behavior Assessment System-3 (ABAS-3) (Harrison & Oakland, 2015)
This is another popular adaptive rating scale which tends to focus on three main areas: the conceptual domains, the social domain, and the practical domain
g. Attention Deficit Hyperactivity Disorder Rating Scales such as the DuPAul ADHD Rating Scale—5 for Children and Adolescents or the Swanson, Nolan and Pelham Teacher and Parent Rating Scale (SNAP-IV)
Other measures of personality and emotional/psychological functioning
a. Beck Youth Inventories-2 (Beck, Beck, Jolly, & Steer, 2005)
The Beck Inventories are five separate self-report behavior rating scales measuring depression, anxiety, anger, disruptive behavior, and self-concept
b. Minnesota Multiphasic Personality Inventory-Adolescent (MMPI-A) (Butcher et al., 1992)
The MMPI-A is considered to be an empirically based measure of adolescent psychopathology
c. Millon Adolescent Clinical Inventory (MACI) (Millon, Millon, & Davis, 1993)
This self-report inventory measures four main areas: personality scales, expressed concerns, clinical syndromes, and modifying indices

Finally, we also offer a caveat here about projective testing. In our clinical experience, children, adolescents, and adults with perceptual processing challenges are not often found in any of the standardization populations for projective tests. Perceptual processing challenges can produce responses on projective instruments that can sometimes be misconstrued as psychopathology. Hence we recommend that they are not used when trying to evaluate and understand clients with NVLD.

6.1 How to Inform Parents About the Results After Testing

First and foremost, as is proposed throughout this book, a parent conference is a psychological/therapeutic event. Indeed the assessment process itself can be viewed as the beginning of treatment. These ideas sometimes called Therapeutic Assessment have been discussed by others in the field (Krishnamurthy, Finn, & Aschieri, 2016). The goals are to establish together a realistic understanding of their child/the client's strengths and challenges, while also providing a measure of hopefulness. Hopelessness is the enemy of progress.

It is very important for parents/caretakers to be encouraged to carefully review their child's evaluation, either as a draft prior to meeting with the evaluator or in a collaborative process together in a meeting, to make sure it accurately captures their child. Does it feel like the evaluator understood the struggles that they were concerned about for their child? If they thought that their child has NVLD but the evaluator did not discuss this, they can use the guidelines for a diagnosis outlined in Chap. 3 to refer to the evaluator in order to try and see if their child might meet diagnostic criteria. At the end of Chap. 7, we list specific tests that we believe should be considered for addition to a battery used to assess for NVLD.

We believe it is best that both parents attend the conference so that they can hear the same thing to try to avoid misunderstandings, as well as each parent getting a chance to ask whatever questions they need to ask. As mentioned above, families are offered the option of receiving a draft report with the test results in the appendix to review prior to the meeting if desired, or they can wait until the meeting to review the report with the evaluator. Second, students should always receive some feedback from the evaluator about their learning profile. Different evaluators do this in different ways, but it is *essential* that students are given age-appropriate feedback about their performance. When people put forth great effort (as is required during a neuropsychological assessment), they must receive feedback; otherwise motivation decreases. In one of our practices (AM), a brief brochure is created specifically for the child, targeted at the correct level for their comprehension, that reviews strengths, weaknesses, and strategies they can use (Fig. 6.1).

This brings up the question of whether the child/adolescent should attend the conference with the parents. The age and maturity of the child is a significant factor in making a recommendation. Our guidance is that the number one priority is that the parents feel free to ask any question they desire without having to worry about how the child is feeling about the question or possible response. However, we are also hoping to engage the child's agency and curiosity regarding how their mind works. So we can provide joint sessions, sessions with parents, then child, then all, and sessions where we have a parent session, a separate child session, and then a joint session individualized to the specific needs of the family.

BROOKLYN LEARNING CENTER

142 Joralemon Street 3E
Brooklyn New York 11201
PHONE 718-935-0400
BrooklynLearningCenter.com

Name: **Date of Feedback:**
Evaluator:

Big picture: You are a smart, hard-working student who learns through verbal channels in low-stress settings

Strengths

- Abstract Verbal reasoning
- Verbal Memory
- Verbal fluency and Idea Generation
- Reading Comprehension

Things for school to provide

- 50% Extra Time on all standardized and in class tests
- Separate room for testing
- Extra time = advanced notice for larger projects or assignments
- Computer for writing assignments
- Calculator for math tests

Weaknesses

- Visual-Spatial Reasoning
- Processing Speed
- Worrying and regulating worry
- Executive Functions: switching, planning

Study Strategies

- Make material verbal – talk it out!
- Elaborate on what you read—make information meaningful
- Follow a writing structure
- Break down assignments into parts
- Use a planner or organize to track time management strategies/plan how long it will take to complete assignments
- Reduce motor demands (e.g., handwriting) when possible—use a computer!

Things to keep on doing

- Keep up your excellent work ethic!
- Ask for extra time so that you can process information and plan your response
- Remember to have fun—make time for low-pressure activities in addition to studying and running!

Fig. 6.1 Model brochures for two middle grade students with NVLD

BROOKLYN LEARNING CENTER

142 Joralemon Street 3E
Brooklyn New York 11201
PHONE 718-935-0400
BrooklynLearningCenter.com

Student: **Feedback Date:**

Big picture: You are a likeable, hardworking student who needs strategies for paying attention and learns best through verbal channels.

Strengths

- Thinking and reasoning with words (Verbal Reasoning)
- Word Knowledge
- Immediate memory for verbal information
- Spelling words
- Writing (when you are told what to do)
- Switching between ideas
- Perseverance and work ethic
- Kind, generous nature

Challenges

- Making sense of novel or visual-spatial information
- Paying attention over time
- Putting information and remembering information in *sequence*
- Getting your great ideas out
- Understanding language that is not straightforward or clear
- Math
- Anxious feelings

Things to keep on doing

- Find the aspects of each subject that interest you and run with it
- Be proud of your hard work, your kind personality, and trust your abilities!
- Remember to keep doing the fun things you love, like soccer

Things for school to provide

- Extra time for tests
- Separate room for tests
- Answer questions directly in test booklet
- Use of a calculator
- Use of a computer when writing and taking notes
- Big tests split up into 2 days

Study Strategies

- Make **priority lists** for homework and start on the **hardest** assignments first
- Clear your homework space of distractions
- Take breaks!
- Make material verbal: Talk it out!
- Use a **timer** when doing homework so you know when to work and when to take breaks
- When **writing**, brainstorm your ideas first, then get your ideas on paper (typing), then organize your ideas, and lastly, edit your work
- When doing math homework, have an **example of the problem** worked out in front of you that shows all of the steps
- You have so many talents- make sure to use supports to your advantage so you can reach your potential and show what you know!

Fig. 6.1 (continued)

6.2 Parent Conference/Feedback Session

We typically start with reviewing two issues: what prompted the referral and what were the main concerns/questions raised by the parents. We then ask for an update on the child and whether any new questions or concerns have emerged. Next, we review the academic data in terms of absolute and relative strengths and challenges sometimes using a normal curve or other visual referents to aid understanding. As we review any of the data, we are also conscious of needing to contextualize the results, such as do they appear to be an accurate reflection of the child's abilities or low or high estimates given how the testing proceeded, i.e., tiredness, heat, motivation, anxiety, etc. The parents should be able to report back on and correct any misconceptions to increase its accuracy and if needed ask for adjustments to be made to the report.

We then review the cognitive data using the same model as above. We help the family understand the relationship and meaning of each score and between the scores and between the different tests. We try to create a shared understanding of why their child was struggling and what their child needs to be most successful. Lastly, we create a plan for the next steps together (see Chap. 10 for the specifics on how to create an action plan).

With respect to NVLD, there are specific ways a student can be supported through school, including accommodations for testing and modification to curriculum. In addition, outside professionals or after-school programs can provide individual support (these are discussed in Chap. 13). All of these ideas are reviewed with parents during the feedback meeting.

It is common for a test report to end with recommendations tailored to the specific child's strengths and weaknesses. A report is a list of specific interventions based on the data gathered on the specific student under question. Then, given the child's profile, the parent's skills/abilities and resources, and the resources within the school and community, the clinician needs to work with the family to prioritize the interventions and accommodations which would be most important for that child at that time. Importantly, the clinician also needs to explain that the specific child's needs are very likely to change over time as the child develops and the interventions enhance the student's coping and learning. An unprioritized "laundry list" is most often overwhelming to a parent and therefore unhelpful. Examples of specific tips for parents and professionals for working with students with NVLD are included in Chap. 7, where we review the process and parts of a neuropsychological evaluation, particularly for children with NVLD, and how to use evaluations to obtain services for children with NVLD.

6.3 Feedback Meeting for Students

The content and format of a feedback meeting for students will vary depending on the student's age and desires, but in general we recommend students be given the choice of having some part of the meeting without their parents present. Figure 6.1 is an example of a model brochure for two different middle grade students with NVLD used by the Brooklyn Learning Center. During this individual portion of the feedback meeting, the evaluator can discuss the child's strengths and difficulties, without use of scores or labels.

We find it helpful to link the information to the child's self-assessment and to begin with strengths. So we usually first review what students did well and easily and how they viewed their own performance. We then discuss difficulties, and we try to tie this to the student's personal experience. For example, we might say, "during the puzzles we did when you had to put blocks together to build a target design, you said: 'this is really hard.' I saw that it was hard for you, but when I gave you a grid to put over the design you were able to solve the puzzles!" Then you can discuss how analogous kinds of strategies can be put into place for students at home during homework, in school, or in social settings. We also provide students with a brochure that outlines their strengths, challenges, and strategies that they use and new ones we recommend to help overcome difficulties. The more specific to each child this can be, the better. If a child has a particular concern at the outset of testing about school, homework, or social activities, it is ideal to provide a strategy or solution for this problem on their feedback brochure.

6.4 Seeking Evaluations for Families with Limited Resources

In our view, this is one of the most difficult challenges facing therapists and professionals who are working with students with NVLD. Generating a well-coordinated treatment approach and treatment team that operates across school and home environments, with group and individual level services delivered during and after school, is extremely important. It also requires a lot of patience, expertise, and perseverance. When families are stressed because children face academic and emotional difficulties, the additional financial stressors associated with supporting a child with special needs can be extremely hard to manage. Our healthcare system does little to help families with limited resources handle any type of health problem; when the problem is viewed as educational, as is the case with learning disabilities, it can be almost impossible for families to access mental health services.

In our clinical experience, we have seen several paths forward for families with limited resources to obtain services for children. The first thing we suggest is that families find an ally at school. This could be the school psychologist, a classroom teacher, or an elective teacher; it just needs to be someone who is invested in helping the child. Even if this person has no influence on policy-making or decision-making power with respect to service delivery, this person can help parents understand the school system, know who to talk to, and try to help make a plan. This person can also advocate on behalf of the student to decision-makers about services they perceive the student to need. When such requests come from adults other than parents, they are often more easily accepted.

The second thing we suggest is do not give up. Continue to ask for what you believe your child needs. If you read about NVLD and believe your child fits this model, request an evaluation to assess the difficulties you observe your child facing; do it in writing. Every child is entitled to an assessment if parents believe that the child is exhibiting problems. Part of the reason children are not assessed is that all parents want to believe that their child is OK, and when they approach skeptical school personnel who say a student is doing OK, they often back away from the request for an assessment.

There is nothing inherently wrong with having a disability and the stigma associated with it is unwarranted. Many children face mental health challenges during their childhood and adolescence. Twenty-two percent of all children in the United States currently have a mental health disorder, and 49% will have a diagnosable mental health problem at some point before the age 18 (Merikangas et al., 2010). Only 14% of children in the United States each year receive special education services (https://nces.ed.gov/programs/coe/indicator_cgg.asp). One take-home message is that families need to feel more empowered to access services for their children. Once the evaluation is completed by the school district, discuss NVLD with the evaluator. Parents and therapists can use the criteria outlined in this book to discuss their views about NVLD with the school personnel.

Last, all parents have the right to request a second, independent educational evaluation (IEE) funded by the school district if you believe the assessment does not address your concerns about your child. There are usually not-for-profit organizations that can help parents request these IEEs if they need help. IEEs are extremely helpful and often correctly identify needed accommodations and services for children. Additionally, parents can obtain compensatory services for children which can address gaps in learning and are often delivered by a provider of the family's choosing, so parents can select a provider who is knowledgeable about NVLD or at least the aspects of it with which a child is struggling. Our hope is that once a clinical definition is accepted in DSM5, more providers will understand NVLD, and it will be easier for families to obtain services within the school and healthcare systems. Tables 6.3 and 6.4 offer low fee assessment resources. The information is culled from the following useful websites (note, there is a focus on services available in the United States):

https://ldaamerica.org/category/assessment-evaluation/assessment-evaluation-for-adults/
https://www.211.org
https://scottishriteforchildren.org/request-appointment
https://www.parentcenterhub.org/find-your-center
https://www.understood.org/en/school-learning/special-services/special-education-basics/parent-training-centers-a-free-resource

Table 6.3 Examples of low cost or sliding scale assessment resources (United States)

Common Examples of Low Cost or Sliding Scale Fee Assessment Resources
Health Insurance If you have health insurance, it's a good idea to contact your insurance company, too. Your policy may cover some or all of the cost of an evaluation. Some types of evaluations may not be covered, though. Most will not pay for assessment for a "learning disability," but they will pay part of the cost of assessment if the need is the result of emotional problems or ADHD. Thus, if a person is depressed and having difficulty at work and the psychologist suspects a learning disability may be an underlying component, assessment can be requested for the depression. Such an assessment would also need to look at cognitive functioning. In this case, if the referral question comes under the DSM-IV Code2 of depression, an insurance company will often help defray costs
Vocational Rehabilitation Services have funds to do assessment. "It is important in this case that the request for assessment clearly links to the possible severity of a learning disability and/or AD/HD to employment. A person, who calls and says, 'I need to be tested for learning disabilities' is likely to be told there are no funds. If the same person says 'I am unable to obtain employment and my counselor said I may have a learning disability,' it is far more likely that funds for testing will be made available." http://www.ldonline.org/article/6021/
Most universities and teaching hospitals that provide graduate training in psychology or school psychology often have clinics that offer low-cost testing and evaluation for learning disabilities for children and adults through their graduate and PhD programs. These clinics are staffed by graduate and PhD candidate students as part of their training under the supervision of an experienced licensed psychologist. They offer evaluations at lower fees or a sliding scale and are free to low-income families. You can contact your local college, university, or a training hospital and ask if they operate a clinic that performs testing evaluations
An advocate who specializes in helping adults with LD and/or ADHD may know of private practitioners in your area who will do low cost, or pro bono, assessment
Psychologists If you call and explain your financial situation, some may provide low-cost assessment. This is the decision of the individual professional.
Your State Special Education or GED Center may have a list of professionals who will provide low-cost assessments
Vocational Rehabilitation Services are an option if the client is headed toward a non-university career
Temporary Assistance for Needy Families (TANF) welfare to work programs (depending upon the issues) may provide assessment services
By law, all evaluations for school-age children are free. Children who are struggling in learning are entitled to an assessment. You can request a free evaluation from your child's school as defined by IDEA (Individuals with Disabilities Education Act

https://www.ldrfa.org/learning-disability-assessment/

Free or Low-Cost Private Evaluations for Learning Disabilities & ADHD-https://www.understood.org/en/family/managing-everyday-challenges/financial-challenges/how-to-get-free-low-cost-evaluation-for-child

The links above are provided for your convenience only and do not imply an endorsement of the information or services provided by listed practitioners. We are unable to provide any warranty regarding the permanence, accuracy, or completeness of the content of such sites or the reliability, quality, or effectiveness of any services provided.

Table 6.4 Additional resources for assessments

Parent Training and Information Centers (PTIs)
Every state has at least one PTI that provides support and information to families funded by the Individuals with Disabilities Education Act (IDEA). Staff at the PTI may be able to suggest where to get a low-cost private evaluation. Some states also have Community Parent Resource Centers, which have more resources for low-income families. Learn how to find a PTI near you. The centers help the families of kids from birth to age 22 who have a disability. The main goal of PTIs is to give parents or guardians support and free information on how to make the most of their child's education. The centers provide families with information about specific disabilities and issues
Community Parent Resource Centers
Some states have community centers in addition to PTIs. The community centers work mainly with low-income families or families that speak English as a second language. These centers make sure parents understand their rights in the special education process. The centers also help families communicate with schools and participate in their child's education. Parent centers offer workshops and training sessions about IDEA, special education, and disabilities. They can also suggest ways at home to help kids who learn and think differently. The centers often have lists of tutors, educational specialists, and special programs or schools. Many centers also have large libraries of helpful books, videos, and pamphlets. Some of this information is available at no cost. Some centers also send out newsletters. Finding a center near you can be a little tricky because the centers go by different names. In some states the names are straightforward, like PTI Nebraska. But New Mexico's PTI is called Parents Reaching Out. A national website called the Center for Parent Information and Resources (CPIR) has a state-by-state listing of PTIs
American Academy of Child and Adolescent Psychiatry (AACAP) ADHD Resource Center
AACAP is a non-profit resource center that provides information and clinical resources for parents. Use their website to find child and adolescent psychiatrists and other mental health professionals in your area
Health Resources and Services Administration (HRSA) Network
HRSA provides a nationwide network of community health centers for families who don't have access to primary healthcare. Finding a center near you can be a good way to look for a low-cost specialist
Scottish Rite Hospital for Children takes referrals for evaluation for learning disorders
211.org This free service connects people with a range of services in their area. In almost every state, you can call 2-1-1 to get easy access to information about health and human services. 211's specialists help evaluate your needs and figure out your options for local programs and services to help
Learning Disabilities Association of America (LDA)
LDA provides information and resources to people with learning disabilities and their families. Each state has a local chapter, and the state affiliates often have referral services available to parents and children. Call and ask if they can help you find low-cost evaluation options in your area
Early Childhood Technical Assistance Center (ECTA Center)

ECTA is the central hub to find the early intervention services in your state. If your baby or toddler is behind other kids in development, visit the ECTA to find out about a free early intervention evaluation. You can also look up the early intervention program in your state
Learning Disability Assessment Resources: ldrfa.org
The Learning Disability National Helpline: 212.645.6730
The National Center for Learning Disabilities: Phone: 212.545.7510 Web: http://www.ld.org/
The Literacy Assistance Center Phone: 212.803.3300 Web: http://www.lacnyc.org/
Check for local resources – For example, in the NYC area the following are possible resources:
Metro New York/New Jersey Learning Disability Evaluation Centers
Adelphi University Center for Psychological Services Office: 1 South Ave., Garden City, NY 11530 Testing Site (no office): 75 Varick St., New York, NY 10013 Phone: 516-877-4820/212.965.8340 Fax: 212.431.5161 https://derner.adelphi.edu/
Beth Israel Medical Center 317 East 17th Street New York, NY 10003 Phone: 212.420.4111
Child Mind Institute 101 East 56th Street New York, NY 10022 Phone: 212.308.3118 Web: https://childmind.org/center/learning-and-development-center/ Offers a program free of cost for participants in research data collection https://childmind.org/center/early-childhood-evaluation/

(continued)

Table 6.4 (continued)

City College Psychological Center
North Academic Center, 8th Fl Room 101 160 Convent Avenue New York, NY 10031 Phone: 212.650.6602 Cost is Low fee or free to low Income $0 https://www.thepsychologicalcenter.org/psychological-assessment/
Columbia University Teachers College Center of Educational and Psychological Services Thorndike Hall 6th floor Box 91 525 West 120th St. New York, NY 10027 Phone: 212.678.3262 Fax: 212.678.8105 https://www.tc.columbia.edu/deanhope/
Fairleigh Dickinson University Center for Psychological Services 131 Temple Avenue Hackensack, NJ 07601 Phone: 201.692.2645 Https://www.fdu.edu
Fisher Landau Center for the Treatment of Learning Disabilities (Albert Einstein) Russo Building 1165 Morris Park Ave. 2nd Floor Bronx, NY 10461 Phone: 718.430.3906 Fax: 718.892.2296 Web: http://www.aecom.yu.edu/cerc/projects.htm#fisher

Fordham University Graduate School of Education Division of Psychological and Educational Services Rosa A. Hagin School Consultation Center 3 West 60th Street, 8th Floor New York, NY 10023 Phone: 212.636.6483 Fax: 212.636.7362 Email: SCECcenters@fordham.edu Reduced Fee https://www.fordham.edu/info/21080/rosa_a_hagin_consultation_and_early_childhood_centers/3235/assessment_procedures_and_fees Sliding scale Fees
Hofstra University Saltzman Community Center Building 1000 Fulton Avenue Hempstead, NY 11549 Phone: 516.463.5660 Web: https://www.hofstra.edu/community/slzctr/slzctr_psych.html
Lenox Hill Hospital Outpatient Center for Mental Health 210 East 64th Street New York, NY 10021 Phone: (212) 838-9200 Web: https://meeth.northwell.edu/center-for-learning-and-attention
Long Island Jewish Medical Center The Zucker Hillside Hospital 75-59 263rd St. Glen Oaks, NY 11004 Phone: 718.470.8763

(continued)

Table 6.4 (continued)

Long Island University, CW Post Campus Psychological Services Center 720 Northern Blvd, Lodge A Brookville, NY 11548 Phone: 516-299-3211 Sliding Scale Fee http://www.liu.edu/CWPost/Academics/College-of-Liberal-Arts-and-Sciences/Doctor-of-Psychology/Psychological-Services-Center
New York Hospital – Cornell Medical Center International Center for the Disabled (ICD) – Learning Disabilities Clinic 340 East 24th St. 6th Floor New York, NY 10010 Phone: 212.585.6240 Fax: 212.585.6161
New York Presbyterian Hospital – Westchester Division 21 Bloomingdale Road White Plains, NY 10605 Phone: 914.997.5776
NYU Medical Center Rusk Institute Learning Diagnostic Center 400 East 34th Street New York, NY 10016 Phone: 212.263.7753 Fax: 212.263.7721
Pace University Dyson College of Arts and Science Thomas J. McShane Center of Psychological Services 156 Williams St. 5th Floor New York, NY 10038 Phone: 212.346.1730 Web: http://appserv.pace.edu/execute/page.cfm?doc_id=5190

Queens College Psychological Center 65-30 Kissena Blvd. New York, NY 11367 Phone: 718.570.0500 https://qcpages.qc.cuny.edu/Psychology/QCPC/index.html Low fee for students with Medical Insurance
Renaissance Health Care Network Developmental Evaluation Clinic 115 West 116th Street New York, NY 10026 Phone: 212.961.5755
Rutgers Psychological Clinic Graduate School of Applied & Professional Psychology 152 Frelinghuysen Road Piscataway, NJ 08854 Phone: 848.445.6111 https://grapple.rutgers.edu/centers-clinical-services/CPS/clinical-services
(The) Sachs Center 235 West 76th Street #1B New York, NY 10023 Phone: 646.807.8900
St. John's University Center for Psychological Services and Clinical Studies Seton Complex, 152-11 Union Turnpike Jamaica, NY 11439 Phone: 718.990.1900/6703 Fax: 718.990.1586

(continued)

Table 6.4 (continued)

Staten Island Jewish Community Center- Learning Institute for Adults 475 Victory Boulevard Staten Island, NY 10301 Phone: 718.987.5542
The Great Kills Psychological Foundation 3915 Hylan Boulevard Staten Island, NY 10308 Phone: 718.948.7800
The J.W. Beatman Counseling Center-The Jewish Board 521 West 239th Street, 3rd Floor Riverdale, NY 10463 Phone: 718.601.7805 Fax: 718.601.7809 Web: https://jewishboard.org/listing/j-w-beatman-counseling-center
Health Resources & Service Administration (HRSA) provides regional health centers for families who don't have access to health insurance or primary healthcare.
Mt. Sinai Adolescent Health Center (ages 10–21) 312 East 94th St. New York, NY Phone: 212.423.3000/212.423.2142 Fee Range: Accept insurance OR all services are free Web: https://www.mountsinai.org/locations/adolescent-health-center/services/learning-disabilities
The JCC-Manhattan 334 Amsterdam Avenue at 76th Street-Lower Level 2 MultiMedia Center New York, NY 10023
CogniTech Cafe AT Support Program Web: http://fhfnyc.org//2013/06/05/cognitech-cafes-free-assistive-technology-support-to-Individuals-with-disabilities/

Next in Chap. 7, we present the common composition of a test report. We offer a guide on the structure of the report, the types of scores presented in the report, and how to interpret and read a test report.

References

Achenbach, T. M., & Rescorla, L. A. (2001). *Manual for the ASEBA school-age forms & profiles*. Burlington, VT: University of Vermont, Research Center for Children, Youth, & Families.

Adams, W., & Sheslow, D. (1995). *Wide range assessment of visual motor abilities manual*. Torrance, CA: Western Psychological Services.

Beck, J. S., Beck, A. T., Jolly, J. B., & Steer, R. A. (2005). *Beck youth inventories second edition for children and adolescents manual*. San Antonio, TX: Psychological Corporation.

Beery, K. E., & Beery, N. A. (2010). *Administration, scoring, and teaching manual for the Beery-VMI* (6th ed.). San Antonio, TX: Pearson. behavior checklist and revised behavior profile. Burlington.

Berninger, V. W. (2007). *Process assessment of the learner-II*. San Antonio, TX: Harcourt Assessment.

Broitman, J., & Davis, J. M. (2013). Treating NVLD in Children: Professional Collaborations for Positive Outcomes.

Brown, J. A., Fishco, V. V., & Hanna, G. (1993). *Nelson–Denny reading test: Manual for scoring and interpretation, forms G & H*. Rolling Meadows, IL: Riverside Publishing.

Butcher, J. N., Williams, C. L., Graham, J. R., Archer, R. P., Tellegen, A., Ben-Porath, Y. S., et al. (1992). *Minnesota multiphasic personality inventory-adolescent version (MMPI-A): Manual for administration, scoring and interpretation*. Minneapolis, MN: University of Minnesota Press.

Carrow-Woolfolk, E. (2017). *Comprehensive assessment of spoken language, second edition (CASL-2) [manual]*. Torrance, CA: Western Psychological Services.

Conners, C. K. (2014). *Conners continuous performance test- third edition (Conners CPT 3) & Conners Continuous Auditory Test of Attention (Conners CATA): Technical manual*. New York: Multi-Health Systems Inc.

Conners, K. C. (2008). *Conners rating scales* (3rd ed.). Toronto, ON: Multi-Health Systems.

Connolly, A. J. (2007). *Key Math Test- 3:Diagnostic Assessment*. San Antonio, TX: Pearson.

Cornoldi, C., Venneri, A., Marconato, F., Molin, A., & Montinari, C. (2003). A rapid screening measure for the identification of visuospatial learning disability in schools. *Journal of Learning Disabilities, 36*(4), 299–306.

Delis, D. C., Kaplan, E., & Kramer, J. H. (2001). *The Delis-Kaplan executive function system*. San Antonio, TX: The Psychological Corporation.

Delis, D. C., Kramer, J. H., Kaplan, E., & Ober, B. A. (1994). *CVLT-C: California verbal learning test*. San Antonio, TX: NCS Pearson.

Dunn, W. (2014). *Sensory profile 2 manual*. San Antonio, TX: Pearson.

Elliot, C. D. (2007). *Differential ability scales* (2nd ed.). San Antonio, TX: Harcourt Assessment.

Feifer, S. G., & Clark, H. K. (2018). *Feifer assessment of math*. Lutz, FL: PAR. Inc.

Gioia, G. A., Isquith, P. K., Guy, S. C., & Kenworthy, L. (2015). *BRIEF2: Behavior rating inventory of executive function* (2nd ed.). Lutz, FL: Psychological Assessment Resources.

Harrison, P., & Oakland, T. (2015). *Adaptive behavior assessment system, third edition (ABAS-3)*. San Antonio, TX: Pearson.

Krishnamurthy, R., Finn, S. E., & Aschieri, F. (2016). Therapeutic assessment in clinical and Counseling psychology practice. *The Wiley handbook of personality assessment* (pp. 228–239). https://doi.org/10.1002/9781119173489.ch17.

Korkman, M., Kirk, U., & Kemp, S. (2007). *NEPSY-II: A developmental neuropsychological assessment*. San Antonio, TX: The Psychological Corporation.

Margolis, A. E., Broitman, J., Davis, J. M., Alexander, L., Hamilton, A., Liao, Z., et al. (2020). Estimated prevalence of nonverbal learning disability among north American children and adolescents. *JAMA Network Open, 3*(4), e202551–e202551. https://doi.org/10.1001/jamanetworkopen.2020.2551

Merikangas, K., Hep, J., Burstein, M., Swanson, S., Avenevoli, S., Cui, L., et al. (2010). Lifetime prevalence of mental disorders in U.S. adolescents: Results from the National Comorbidity Survey Replication—Adolescent Supplement (NCS-A). *Journal of American Academy of Child and Adolescent Psychiatry., 49*(10), 980–989. https://doi.org/10.1016/j.jaac.2010.05.017

Meyers, J. E., & Meyers, K. R. (1995). *Rey complex figure test and recognition trial.* Odessa, FL: Psychological Assessment Resources.

Millon, T., Millon, C., & Davis, R. (1993). *Millon adolescent clinical inventory manual.* Minneapolis, MN: National Computer Systems.

Phelps-Terasaki, D., & Phelps-Gunn, T. (1992). *Test of pragmatic language* (2d ed.). Torrance, CA: Western Psychological Services.

Reynolds, C. R., & Kamphaus, R. W. (2015). *Behavior assessment for children: Third edition. (BASC-3).* Bloomington, MN: Pearson.

Richman, J. E., & Garzia, R. P. (2015). The Developmental Eye Movement Test. Mishawaka: IN. Bernell Corporation.

Richman, Connolly, A. J. (2007). Key Math Test-3: Diagnostic Assessment. San Antonio, TX: Pearson, and J. E. & Garzia, R. P. (2015). The Developmental Eye Movement Test. Mishawaka: IN. Bernell Corporation.

Sandson, T. A., Bachna, K. J., & Morin, M. D. (2000). Right hemisphere dysfunction in ADHD: Visual hemispatial inattention and clinical subtype. *Journal of Learning Disabilities, 33*(1), 83–90. https://doi.org/10.1177/002221940003300111

Sheslow, D., & Adams, W. (2003). *Wide range assessment of memory and learning: Second edition- administration and technical manual.* Lutz, FL: Psychological Assessment Resources.

Sparrow, S. S., Cicchetti, D. V., & Saulnier, C. A. (2016). *Vineland adaptive behavior scales, third edition (Vineland-3).* San Antonio, TX: Pearson.

Torgesen, J. K., Wagner, R. K, & Rashotte, C. A. (2012). *Test of word reading efficiency* (2nd Ed.). (*TOWRE-2*). Austin, TX: Pro-Ed.

Wagner, R. K., Torgesen, J. K., Rashotte, C. A., & Pearson, N. A. (2013). *Comprehensive test of phonological processing–second edition.* Austin, TX: PRO-ED.

Wechsler, D. (2008). *Wechsler Adult Intelligence Scale* (4th ed.). San Antonio, TX: NCS Pearson.

Wechsler, D. (2009). *Wechsler individual achievement test third edition.* San Antonio, TX: NCS Pearson.

Wechsler, D. (2011). *Wechsler abbreviated scale of intelligence–second edition.* San Antonio, TX: NCS Pearson.

Wechsler, D. (2014). *Wechsler intelligence scale for children-fifth edition.* San Antonio, TX: NCS Pearson.

Wechsler, D., & Naglieri, J. A. (2006). *Wechsler nonverbal scales of intelligence.* San Antonio, TX: Psychological Corporation.

Wiederholt, J. L., & Bryant, B. R. (2012). *Gray oral reading tests – Fifth edition.* Austin, TX: ProEd.

Wiig, E., Semel, E., & Secord, E. (2013). *Clinical evaluation of language fundamentals* (5th ed.). Bloomington, MN: NCS Pearson.

https://ldaamerica.org/where-can-i-go-for-low-cost-or-free-evaluation-services/, https://ldaamerica.org/category/assessment-evaluation/assessment-evaluation-for-adults/

https://www.211.org

Request Appointment https://scottishriteforchildren.org/request-appointment

Find Your Parent Center. Center for Parent Information and Resources https://www.parentcenterhub.org/find-your-center

What Are Parent Training and Information Centers (PTIs)? https://www.understood.org/en/schoollearning/special-services/special-educationbasics/parent-training-centers-a-free-resource

Learning Disability Assessment Resources https://www.ldrfa.org/learning-disability-assessment/

Free or Low-Cost Private Evaluations for Learning Disabilities & ADHD https://www.understood.org/en/family/managingeveryday-challenges/financial-challenges/how-to-getfree-low-cost-evaluation-for-child

Chapter 7
Reading and Interpreting the Neuropsychological Assessment Report

In this chapter we review the process and parts of a neuropsychological evaluation particularly for children with NVLD, how to use evaluations to obtain services for children with NVLD, and finally how to use existing evaluations to retrospectively assess if a person might meet criteria for NVLD.

7.1 The Process and Parts of a Neuropsychological Assessment

When consulting with families and other professionals who are part of the treatment team for children with NVLD, we are often asked how we interpret the neuropsychological test data, what a particular test measures, and how we use the assessment to help with differential diagnosis, recommendations, and treatment planning.

First, we explain that we gather different kinds of information in a neuropsychological evaluation. We collect information through interviews, observations, and test performance. All of these types of information can be used in a norm-referenced process wherein a child's behavior (observed or reported by parents or teachers or on a test administered by a psychologist) is compared to that of their same age peers or behaviors are considered in light of some threshold or guideline for when a particular behavior or set of behaviors reaches "clinical significance." For example, attention deficit hyperactivity disorder (ADHD) is assessed by examining an individual's behavior and by noting to what extent they display the hallmark behaviors of ADHD: hyperactivity, impulsivity, and distractibility. Deficits in attention on cognitive testing help describe the individual and their particular challenges but are not specified in the diagnostic criteria as defined by DSM5. Similarly, our definition for developmental visual–spatial disorder (DVSD) should allow clinicians to use interview formats to elicit information about a person's visual–spatial deficits, which should be complemented by available psychological testing.

J. Broitman et al., *NVLD and Developmental Visual-Spatial Disorder in Children*, https://doi.org/10.1007/978-3-030-56108-6_7

Assessments typically gather information about current and past functioning (developmental, psychiatric, medical, academic) using open-ended interview formats. To ascertain current levels of behavioral difficulties, evaluators use non-standardized tools like open-ended interview formats and classroom observations. In addition, we use standardized assessment tools like behavior rating scales such as the BRIEF-2 or semi-structured clinical interviews such as the Kiddie Schedule for Affective Disorders and Schizophrenia to begin to understand the "presenting problem" that is the reason that prompted an assessment. Once we have collected data from these various sources, we integrate information from a patient's history (development, family history, educational history), collateral sources, performance-based measures, and behavioral observations to provide a narrative about a child's strengths and weaknesses that is linked to specific recommendations. This should make it clear that a neuropsychological assessment is not simply psychometric testing.

We commonly assess a number of domains of functioning, and these contribute to the format of the report. Report structures vary but generally always include (1) medical and educational history; (2) behavior observations in the clinic and in school (preferably weaved in throughout a report and explaining particular results or impressions rather than as a stand-alone section); (3) testing data which is generally structured by cognitive area (as reviewed in Chap. 5: intellectual functioning, executive function, language, etc.); (4) diagnostic impressions that integrate behavioral observations, interview data, and test results; (5) specific referrals, recommendations, and a guide for developing a treatment plan; and (6) technical data, presented either in an appendix or throughout the report.

The individual test performance data will likely be presented in a table. Comprehensive texts on psychological assessment and tests and measurement provide in-depth reviews of the technical properties of test construction and scores. Here we give a brief overview geared toward allowing the reader to review existing neuropsychological assessments for the presence of NVLD. A "raw score" is the individual's actual score on a task, and in order to be meaningful, it must be considered in the context of performance of other individuals, their age or sex, etc. Depending on the measure, these raw scores are converted to standard, scaled, or T scores (mean = 100 standard deviation = 15, mean = 10 standard deviation = 3, mean = 50 standard deviation = 10, respectively). These standardized scores also can be converted to percentiles, which provide an index of where a child falls relative to 100 comparison individuals, i.e., a 63rd percentile means a child performed well or better than 63% of children in the comparison sample. Scores can also be converted to provide age- or grade-equivalent scores, giving a sense of how a student performed relative to the expected level for someone in their age level or grade.

7.2 Services and Support

As mentioned above the assessment report can be used to generate school-based accommodations, support, and modifications to curriculum. These related services are protected under the Individuals with Disabilities Education Act (IDEA) which ensures all students with a disability are eligible for a free and appropriate public education (FAPE) if they need special education. In order to access these services, students need to be classified as having a special education need. The guidelines vary by state, but generally this requires an Individual Educational Plan (IEP) that is determined at a committee on special education (CSE) meeting. This can be very hard to obtain for students with NVLD as the diagnosis is not yet recognized in DSM5 nor are the functional consequences of visual–spatial deficits always acknowledged in school settings. As mentioned in Chap. 2, a new diagnosis and application to DSM5 for inclusion are underway; one motivating factor is to increase access to services for students with NVLD.

Alternatively, students can usually more easily obtain a 504 Plan, which is generated through the Eligibility Laws – Section 504 and ADA. This part of the law protects individuals from discrimination but does not entitle an individual to services. It provides individuals with certain accommodations to ensure *access* to education but does not provide modification to curriculum. There are state-specific guidelines about district responsibilities and deadlines for holding IEP meetings, etc. The school's psychologist should be able to help parents learn their rights in a particular district or state. However, all of the authors have worked with families from around the country who have been met with skepticism and rejection when they have asked for services for their children with NVLD. There are always independent groups such as Advocates for Children or local special education lawyers who can help guide families to the due process laws in their state.

Many services are available to students with disabilities including:

- Integrated Co-Teaching Class (ICT)
- Speech therapy (ST)
- Occupational therapy (OT)
- Transportation
- Assistive technology (AT)
- Push-in service
- Pull-out service
- Classroom accommodations
- Curriculum modification
- Testing accommodations
- Paraprofessional (crisis, health, bus para)
- Bilingual services
- FM unit
- Scribe
- Special Education Teacher Support Services (SETSS)
- Adaptive Physical Education (APE)
- Physical Therapy (PT)

Many of these are quite important for students with NVLD and should be accessed whenever possible. All schools must provide IEP supports, but the manner or location varies by type of school:

- Community school – all/most services at school site

- Charter school – *most* services provided at school site (ST/OT/APE at times provided outside)
- Parochial – many services provided outside of school setting
- Approved non-public school (NPS) – *all* services provided at school setting
- Non-approved non-public school – *all* services provided at school setting
- Other (e.g., Montessori schools) – most services provided at school site (ST/OT/APE at times provided outside)

The IEP is by definition individualized. It establishes educational goals for eligible students for a period of one school year. It is created at a meeting with an IEP Team from the CSE. During these meetings with the student with NVLD in mind, it is particularly important to think about the classification (learning disabled, other health impaired, etc.). This will vary based on the student's particular profile (NVLD subtype), and the most prominent deficits are generally used for making classification, in part because NVLD is not in and of itself a recognized diagnosis. The IEP will also identify a student's levels of functioning, services being provided and the goals for services (academic, behavioral, etc.), testing/classroom accommodations, modifications to curriculum, promotion criteria, and school placement. Parents of children with NVLD and their advocates need to make sure that the services on the IEP are appropriate to NVLD and that the specific needs of individuals with NVLD are met in the IEP.

School placement is often a difficult decision addressed during IEP meetings. All parents hope that their children will be functioning well enough to attend a "regular" education program. Even when parents see their children in distress on a daily basis, parents are likely to let their hope that a regular setting can provide a free and appropriate education (FAPE) cloud their willingness to demand an appropriate setting. It is also challenging (and expensive) to find a school dedicated to educating children with NVLD although there are several models emerging. We believe part of the reason there are so few schools for children with NVLD (e.g., versus dyslexia) is its under-recognition in the diagnostic nomenclature. Schools like Mary McDowell School in Brooklyn, NY; Winston Preparatory in NY, Connecticut, and California; and The Winchendon School in Brooklyn and Massachusetts all have programs designed specifically for students with NVLD. See Chap. 9 for an additional discussion regarding choosing the best learning environment for a child with NVLD.

Parents are entitled to disagree with the decisions of the CSE and placement offer. There are several ways to handle this. Mediation allows the parties to enter into a dialogue about the conflict and reach a mutually agreeable solution. An impartial third person (a trained mediator) facilitates communication between the parties. The parties control the outcome. Instead, the parties may use the process of impartial hearing. This is a legal procedure that takes place within the department of education setting. An impartial hearing officer (IHO) presides over the process and gives both parties the opportunity to present testimony and witnesses. The IHO produces a written document with the findings of fact and the decision based on the evidence. The decision may be appealed. It should also be noted that each of these approaches has financial implications. During the initial IEP, if all agree, the school district is required to absorb all costs for placements and interventions. In mediation there can be cost sharing with the district picking up part of the cost and the parents or guardians picking up part of the costs. Finally, in the impartial hearing, the district must again pay all of the fees/costs associated with the IEP.

Over the years we have collected tips for advocacy for parents that are particularly important for parents of children with NVLD. These families often face the added burden of having to prove that NVLD is a disability, or that the associated features are evidence of a disabling condition, in addition to proving that their child meets the criteria for special education, placement, services, etc. When parents request meetings, they must put it in writing. If a request is not in writing, it never happens. Get to know your IEP team. Get contact information for everyone (all service providers).

Create an email/snail mail/paper trail of requests and conversations about the child's needs. Make sure the challenges that a provider sees that a child faces is in writing before the meeting if possible. Follow up with service providers as much as possible without becoming a burden. Ask at school how you should request services, in writing. Send follow-up notes and "Thank you" emails. If you are requesting a psychoeducational evaluations/re-evaluations, make sure you request this in writing and include information about NVLD.

Show the team the recent paper documenting the prevalence of NVLD at 3–4% of children in the United States. Written requests should be submitted to the school's psychologist and principal. If you are unsure about a school following through on the request, submit the letter to the CSE representative as well. If related services are not being provided, notify the school-based support team (school psychologist/teacher/service provider) and the school principal. Services not provided are owed to a child, and parents can request compensatory services (during school year, summer, or in New York, a Related Service Authorization letter to be provided in the home setting).

7.3 Strategies for Parents and Professional for Working with Students with NVLD

It is important for parents, teachers, and treatment professionals to recognize that there may sometimes be limitations in the child/adolescent's visual, perceptual, and/or sensory processing neural circuitry. They may be less "in sync" whenever material is presented in a way that forces the child to break down and learn new material without any context or accompanying verbal instruction. Therefore, instructions with visual tasks should also be verbally broken down in a logical step-by-step fashion and delivered in an explicit, direct instruction fashion. When something is presented in a visual or multimodal format, it should be accompanied by verbal cues and/or explanations. Instruction needs to be at a pace the learner can keep up with, and more repetition of material is usually required. In particular, we need to keep in mind that the geometric math's and sciences will be particularly difficult for students with NVLD. A student with NVLD will most likely appreciate and benefit from, not tire of, lengthy concrete verbal instructions and/or examples. Verbal mediation is a powerful tool for them. Rely on their verbal strengths to teach decision-making, goal setting, and making action plans to achieve goals and evaluate results.

Likewise, the child/adolescent may have difficulty "seeing the big picture" or the context from which details are extracted. While most people take a whole-part-whole approach to learning novel material, children and adolescents with these issues tend to take a part-whole approach whereby they can become easily stuck in the details. The child can be overwhelmed by large amounts of materials; thus information should be presented in small "chunks" whenever possible. Large amounts of material, information, and homework assignments that have not been structured for the student may be counterproductive given that they could become overwhelmed and distractible when challenged in that way.

The child/adolescent's tendency to get stuck in the details can be anxiety provoking, and the cycle may tend to escalate once it starts. One way to deal with escalating frustration is to teach the child to utilize relaxation techniques that can be used immediately when the frustration cycle begins. Explore with the child which of the many interventions work best for them. Examples of these techniques can be found in Chap. 13. Once the child/adolescent masters any of these techniques, they can be taught to transfer these new skills to other situations that cause him/her anxiety or distress. Further, once relaxed, they can better learn to switch strategies and take an alternative strategy to a novel situation.

The child/adolescent's nonverbal weaknesses can sometimes precipitate social difficulties and possible misperceptions. They may have trouble reading nonverbal cues, especially when they are subtle, and may have difficulty knowing how to respond in novel social situations. It is important to understand that the child may not accurately perceive the "gestalt" in social situations as well and might require explicit direct instruction in this arena as well. They will likely do better in more highly structured social situations, but social skills training can help to better adapt to less structured situations. This training includes a collection of practices that use a behavioral approach for teaching age-appropriate social skills and competencies, including communication, problem-solving, decision-making, self-management, and peer relations. Programs to consider are included in the appendix.

As in most new learning situations, it will also be useful here to anticipate the situations where students with NVLD might have difficulty with transitions or novelty and prepare them by providing advanced practice and support for how to deal with these situations. Don't assume you are seeing a "character flaw" or "bad behavior," instead understand that students with NVLD often misunderstand or miscommunicate their ideas, so try to explore the underlying reasons for their behavior with an open mind.

Try to make the demands for performance as reasonable as possible, i.e., make sure demands are not overwhelming and preview, teach, and practice organizational skills. Utilize structure, routine, and rote or "scripted" rules when necessary to help the child/adolescent better manage situations. Teach the child/adolescent to attend to and interpret facial expressions, gestures, prosody, vocal inflections, and other nonverbal aspects of communication. Help them learn how to self-monitor their progress. There are many different techniques to do this included in the intervention Chap. 15.

7.4 Using Extant Data to Determine If an Individual Meets Criterion for NVLD

We have frequently been asked by professionals in our field and in other fields if one can reinterpret existing neuropsychological data from an individual to make a retrospective NVLD diagnosis. Assessing an individual and understanding if they meet criteria for a disorder requires more than test scores. It requires a holistic understanding of the individual's developmental trajectory, current strengths and difficulties, and functional impairments. In our opinion, professionals who are trained in making this type of assessment can reevaluate extant test data to determine if NVLD is a reasonable diagnosis. Parents are often not trained to make these diagnoses but can instead review a child's assessment and developmental history for the hallmark signs of NVLD and then contact a professional for help moving forward and determining an appropriate diagnosis.

We recommend that parents and professionals follow the method we use in our paper estimating the prevalence of NVLD from extant data. We have developed an algorithm that could determine whether an individual met criteria for NVLD based solely on test scores. Below in Table 7.1, criteria for a provisional NVLD diagnosis, and Table 7.2, specific measures used to make a provisional diagnosis, we list out the steps for making the "provisional" determination and show a table of tests we used because they were available in each data set.

Table 7.1 Criteria for provisional NVLD diagnosis

	Domain	Evidence
Step 1	Visual–spatial deficit	Performance at or below 16th percentile on visual–spatial tests *or* significant discrepancy between verbal and spatial abilities (e.g., VIQ-PIQ≥15 points)
AND	Intact word reading	Performance >16th percentile
Step 2	Social skills Executive function skills Math skills Motor skills	Deficit in at least 2/4 areas Performance ≤ 16th percentile
Step 3	Absence of ASD features	ASD features ruled out by survey or by study exclusion criteria

Note. *ASD* autism spectrum disorder, *VIQ* Verbal Intelligence Quotient, *PIQ* Performance Intelligence Quotient. Originally published in Margolis et al. Estimated Prevalence of Nonverbal Learning Disability Among North American Children and Adolescents. *JAMA Network Open*. 2020;3(4)

Table 7.2 Specific measures used to make a provisional diagnosis

Domain							
	Step 1		Step 2				Step 3
Sample	Spatial deficit	Word reading	Social	EF	Math	Motor	ASD Feature
HBN	WISC/WASI/WAIS MR or BD ≤ 16th percentile OR WISC 5 VIQ-PIQ OR VIQ-FRI > 15 points OR WAIS/WASI VCI-PRI > 15	WIAT Word reading ≥16th percentile	CBCL social problems T ≥70	NIH flaker or card sort ≤ 16th percentile	WIAT Numerical operations ≤ 16th percentile	Grooved Pegboard ≤16th percentile	ASSQ <19
NKI	WASI MR or BD ≤16th percentile OR VIQ-PIQ > 15 points	WIAT Word reading ≥16th percentile	CBCL social problems ≥95th percentile	DKEFS trail making, card sort ≤ 16th percentile	WJ-III Calculation ≤16th percentile	Perdue Pegboard ≤16th percentile	ASD is exclusion for the study
SYS	WISC -III PIQ ≤ 16th percentile OR VIQ-PIQ > 15 points	WJ spelling ≥ 16th percentile	Positive youth development scale ≤ 16th percentile	Stroop interference ≤16th percentile	WJ-III calculation ≤16th percentile	Grooved Pegboard ≤16th percentile	ASD is exclusion for the study

Originally published in Margolis et al. Estimated Prevalence of Nonverbal Learning Disability Among North American Children and Adolescents. *JAMA Network Open*. 2020;3(4)

Similarly, the measures listed in Chap. 6 are organized by domain and can be used for making a provisional determination. In the case of an individual person, their developmental history and current functioning should also be considered. We recommend consulting with a psychologist who has expertise in NVLD to help with this process. In Chap. 8, we address the need for early assessment and accurate treatment for our children with NVLD.

Reference

Margolis, A. E., et al. (2020). Estimated prevalence of nonverbal learning disability among North American children and adolescents. *The Journal of the American Medical Associtation Network Open, 3*(4), e202551.

Chapter 8
The Need for Early Assessment and Accurate Treatment

8.1 The Need for Early Identification

Like many neurodevelopmental disorders, NVLD presents in a variety of ways. In our view NVLD symptoms occur along a spectrum from mild to severe based on the number and severity of symptoms, similar to ADHD. Children may have seemingly mild symptoms and behaviors consistent with NVLD, but may not show a specific functional impairment. Alternatively, they may have enough implicit support in the environment that they do not require formal intervention. In these cases, they will not typically require formal assessment or treatment, since they are not experiencing functional difficulties. Importantly, our clinical observations suggest that overall intellectual potential can mitigate aspects of the challenges that children or adults with NVLD confront, meaning that the lack of functional impairment does not mean that no intervention is indicated.

Supporting these clinical observations, our recent empirical work suggests that within a community sample of children, a high overall Full Scale IQ score can moderate associations between verbal/visual–spatial discrepancies and anxiety, social problems, attention, and executive function (Margolis et al., 2015). The protection or buffer provided by a higher Full Scale IQ may be one reason that some individuals with NVLD are not diagnosed and therefore not treated as early as possible, potentially leading to greater difficulties as they mature than they would have confronted with earlier intervention. Presumably this protection is afforded through higher verbal IQ and reasoning abilities associated with higher overall IQ. Put another way, the enhanced verbal abilities which are often present in NVLD may make it harder to detect underlying impairment, which is nonetheless present.

Psychological and neuropsychological factors influence learning and are influenced by learning problems. Thus we believe that learning problems require psychological intervention as early as possible. It has long been known that early intervention for language delay and language-based learning disorders such as

J. Broitman et al., *NVLD and Developmental Visual-Spatial Disorder in Children*, https://doi.org/10.1007/978-3-030-56108-6_8

reading disorder (dyslexia) improves children's trajectories (DSM5). If problems can be identified early, intervention can begin early, possibly stemming the unfolding of a negative developmental trajectory. For example, the co-occurrence of anxiety and reading problems has long been recognized by teachers and parents. Studies show that anxiety influences children's achievement (Everson, Smodlaka, & Tobias, 1994), that reading problems have a negative influence on anxiety (Carroll, Maughan, Goodman, & Meltzer, 2005), and that children with reading disorder are at increased risk for anxiety symptoms (Greenham, 1999; Margari et al., 2013).

The co-occurrence of reading problems and anxiety is thought to be bidirectional, wherein reading difficulties lead to anxiety symptoms, which in turn lead to continued difficulty reading, or, put the other way, anxiety problems lead to difficulty with reading which in turn gives rise to more anxiety (Grills-Taquechel, Fletcher, Vaughn, & Stuebing, 2012; Ialongo, Edelsohn, Werthamer-Larsson, Crockett, & Kellam, 1995). Moreover, we have shown that children with a reading disorder who *did not have an anxiety disorder* reported higher levels of self-reported anxiety than their typically developing peers and, importantly, showed positive rather than negative connectivity between the amygdala and medial prefrontal cortex (Davis, Margolis, Thomas, Huo, & Marsh, 2018), closely mirroring the neural signature of pediatric anxiety disorder (Qin et al., 2014). Most relevant to treatment implications, we showed that anxiety symptoms are on the causal pathway to reading problems. In short, children with reading disorder *who did not have anxiety disorder* showed the neurobiological and behavioral markers of anxiety problems. These symptoms require early identification and psychological treatment in order to fully address the needs of children with all learning disorders.

Similarly, deficits in executive functions have been reported in children with reading disorder for many years, and these problems are associated with children's reading problems (Bednarek et al., 2004; Booth, Boyle, & Kelly, 2010; Borella, Carretti, & Pelegrina, 2010; Facoetti & Turatto, 2000; Kibby, Lee, & Dyer, 2014; Mahe, Doignon-Camus, Dufour, & Bonnefond, 2014; Purvis & Tannock, 2000; Varvara, Varuzza, Sorrentino, Vicari, & Menghini, 2014; Willcutt et al., 2001; Willcutt, Pennington, Olson, Chhabildas, & Hulslander, 2005). Our recent study documents the difficulty that children with reading disorder have with cognitive control, a specific executive function that can be intervened on in the preschool years (Rosas, Espinoza, Porflitt, & Ceric, 2019). Such work suggests again the importance of *early* and *psychological* intervention for all children with learning disorders including NVLD.

Similar to reading disorder, our clinical experiences suggest that earlier and more accurate diagnosis, coupled with early intervention, yields better outcomes for children with NVLD (Martin, 2007; Thompson, 1997). However, we still have little validated information about how to best treat a visual–spatial deficit and even less about how treatment in the toddler and preschool years improves developmental outcomes for a child with NVLD. It is our hope that future studies will successfully identify the early life behavioral markers of visual–spatial deficits and test interventions in randomized controlled trials in order to validate and identify interventions.

Until this occurs we struggle to do our best with the interventions that have anecdotally appeared to offer success.

8.2 Beginning Treatment

Diagnosis and understanding in hand, it is now time to begin treatment. Evidence suggests that since approximately 65–75% of meaning is communicated by nonverbal cues, such as tone of voice, facial expression, posture, and body language, there is potential for a significant difficulty in pragmatic communications for the child who cannot decipher or interpret nonverbal behavior (Mehrabian, 1971; Nowicki & Duke, 1992; Thompson, 1997). Children with NVLD are at high risk for a multitude of clinical concerns including depression, anxiety disorders, social challenges, and academic issues (Margolis et al., 2019, Rourke, 1988; Semrud-Clikeman, Walkowiak, Wilkinson, & Minne, 2010).

Rourke (1988) argued that untreated, the NVLD profile represents a sufficient condition for the development of psychopathology. He noted that these children are at risk specifically for the development of what he called "internalizing" psychopathology (i.e., depression and anxiety). He theorized that this occurs when the child's nonverbal deficiencies (poor visual spatial, tactile–perceptual, psychomotor, and concept formation skills) and the child's overreliance on verbal skills (resulting in a parroting, repetitive style of speech) interfere with the development of social competency. He hypothesized that such reduced social competency would lead to isolation, low self-esteem, and the onset of depression and anxiety. Multiple studies confirmed those concerns (Semrud-Clikeman, Walkowiak, Wilkinson, & Gina, 2010; Semrud-Clikeman, Fine, & Bledsoe, 2010; Ozonoff, Rogers, & Hendren, 2003; Rourke, 2000; Peck, 1985). Most researchers and practitioners express considerable concern regarding potential for developing future problems and agreement on the need for early intervention (Rourke, Young, & Leenaars, 1989; Semrud-Clikeman, Fine, & Bledsoe, 2010; Peck, 1985).

What, how, and when to treat are complex clinical decisions. The primacy of issues varies with the child's developmental level, as well as the individual strengths and deficits of the child with whom one is working. The family's means and resources must also be considered. As the potential areas of need cross over into many disciplines, a variety of professionals are likely to be involved in what would have to evolve to be a collaborative team model. As we discuss below, a team coordinator or case manager is needed to keep all parties informed regarding the coordination of intervention services as well as the child's progress. A school psychologist would be in a good position to take this role; however anyone might be so designated, including a parent. Thus, the successful treatment of a child with NVLD requires an interactive coordinated team. Let us begin with a review of some general organizing principles that could be of help guiding a team with any psychological orientation toward a successful collaboration.

8.3 General (Non Theory Specific) Intervention Guidelines

One of the practitioner's most important tasks is to help the child and family understand that the child is not the disability. Children with NVLD, like all children, have strengths and weaknesses. It is crucial to help the child learn to understand and best use their unique mind. Many have supported this notion calling it islands of competencies (Brooks, 1991; Brooks & Goldstein, 2001), multiple intelligences (Gardner, 1999), and the eight learning systems that show that "Different minds learn differently" (Levine, 2002) to mention a few. The general rule is that the practitioner must help the child understand and know what their strengths are and how they can be brought to bear on the issue at hand. Whatever areas of strength emerge should be used as a vehicle for helping the child develop and maintain a strong sense of self-competency. In order to help keep these children motivated, we have to incorporate the child's passions into the treatment intervention plan in every way possible. Whoever is involved with the child must focus on achieving the following: Interventions should be direct and explicit (Ahearn, 2010), and they must involve the child and consist largely of verbal communication and modeling (Foss, 1991; Rourke, 1995).

Palombo (2006), a clinical social worker on the staff of the Rush NeuroBehavioral Center in Chicago, who views children with NVLD from a self-psychological perspective, suggests that professionals should focus on interventions that increase the child's coping capacities and improve self-esteem. He believes that children with NVLD face many difficulties, including being socially disconnected and awkward, and are often teased and rejected. He believes this is primarily due to a lack of social competencies. He has observed that children with NVLD struggle to initiate conversation, tend to follow conventional scripts, and have difficulty establishing empathy with peers, matching other's social skills, conceptualizing alternative scenarios, and using cause and effect reasoning, and they struggle with decoding social behavior. He believes that this is due in part to a mind-blindness using Baron-Cohen's (1997) conceptualization for children with ASD or a "theory of mind" problem with attributing mental states to oneself and others resulting in a difficulty making sense and predicting the behavior of others. He further suggests that these problems may be due to both receptive and expressive pragmatic language issues and executive function deficits.

Interventions should reflect an ecological approach to the biopsychosocial needs of the child with NVLD, with an interdisciplinary team of specialists (Little, 1999). Children with NVLD need proper diagnosis, and typically a child neuropsychologist or school psychologist can provide this service. In addition, these children often need assessment by a developmental pediatrician or child psychiatrist for medication evaluation. Medications may help some of the behavioral or psychiatric difficulties, referred to above, that are often comorbid with NVLD. Many children with NVLD are treated with stimulants for attentional issues, and moderate improvement from medication has been documented (Gross-Tsur et al., 1995; Rourke, 1995; Voeller, 1995). Antidepressants have also been used for anxiety and depression, and there is some clinical documentation of trials with mood stabilizers as well (Ternes, Woody, & Livingston, 1987). Little (1999) further suggests that children with NVLD need Individualized Educational Plans (IEP) if they are in the public schools, or treatment plans if not, that take into account the nature of their deficits and strengths. This will include modifications, accommodations, and strategies to teach them the skills they need to develop (Thompson, 1997).

A primary aid to the child's learning is to teach him or her sequentially and to use the child's verbal strengths to compensate for weaknesses whenever possible. The child will need training in social skills and pragmatics; these skills are not part of a general education curriculum or typical education plan. In addition children with NVLD often need assistance with reading comprehension. Active reading strategies such as pre-reading, chunking, paraphrasing, and self-quizzing can be effective for improving comprehension. It may also be beneficial to have the child read out loud, concurrently with other active reading strategies. For example, orally pre-reading a textbook chapter or orally processing a visual aid in a textbook may trigger and/or increase understanding. Instructional efforts that help generate clear meanings can improve comprehension. A step-by-step, parts-to-whole teaching approach may help broaden perspective and increase recognition. This is because students with NVLD may focus only on small parts of an assignment while neglecting the larger picture (Foss, 1991). These small segments may be the baseline of comprehension, and, due to problem-solving deficits, it becomes necessary for the teacher to break down their lessons into microunits. It is essential that assumptions regarding ability not be made and that this step-by-step approach starts where the student's skills begin to break down.

There is considerable overlap and agreement across disciplines. All agree with meeting the child where they are, scaffolding the intervention to plan for success, and removing the scaffolding slowly when convinced that the child has internalized the lessons. Verbal mediation is seen by all as the most likely key strategy for helping the child encode the necessary lessons. Agreement exists that one must make sure that the plan for success includes planning for generalization and transfer of the skills from the clinician's office to the real worlds of home, school, playground, and community. As NVLD is a developmental disability, the child's needs constantly shift and change as the child matures. Providers must do the same, creating individualized, age appropriate treatment plans. Treating a child or adult with NVLD requires a team with many supporting players. It is imperative that all of the providers work from compatible theoretical perspectives regarding how patients learn, develop, and change. What follows in Chap. 9 is a discussion regarding the importance of working from a shared theoretical orientation and our team's psychological orientation for treatment.

References

Baron-Cohen, S. (1997). *Mindblindness: An essay on autism and theory of mind*. Cambridge, MA: MIT press.

Bednarek, D. B., Saldana, D., Quintero-Gallego, E., Garcia, I., Grabowska, A., & Gomez, C. M. (2004). Attentional deficit in dyslexia: A general or specific impairment? *Neuroreport, 15*(11), 1787–1790.

Booth, J. N., Boyle, J. M., & Kelly, S. W. (2010). Do tasks make a difference? Accounting for heterogeneity of performance of children with reading difficulties on tasks of executive function: Findings from a meta-analysis. *British Journal of Developmental Psychology, 28*(Pt 1), 133–176.

Borella, E., Carretti, B., & Pelegrina, S. (2010). The specific role of inhibition in reading comprehension in good and poor comprehenders. *Journal of Learning Disabilities, 43*(6), 541–552. https://doi.org/10.1177/0022219410371676.

Brooks, R. (1991). *The self-esteem teacher*. Loveland, OH: Treehaus Communications.

Brooks, R., & Goldstein, S. (2001). *Raising resilient children: Fostering strength, Hope, and optimism in your child*. Lincolnwood, IL: Contemporary Books.

Carroll, J. M., Maughan, B., Goodman, R., & Meltzer, H. (2005). Literacy difficulties and psychiatric disorders: Evidence for comorbidity. *Journal of Child Psychology and Psychiatry, and Allied Disciplines, 46*(5), 524–532. https://doi.org/10.1111/j.1469-7610.2004.00366.x.

Davis, K., Margolis, A. E., Thomas, L., Huo, Z., & Marsh, R. (2018). Amygdala sub-regional functional connectivity predicts anxiety in children with reading disorder. *Developmental Science, 21*(5), e12631–e12631. https://doi.org/10.1111/desc.12631.

Everson, H. T., Smodlaka, I., & Tobias, S. (1994). Exploring the relationship of test anxiety and metacognition on reading test performance: A cognitive analysis. *Anxiety, Stress, and Coping, 7*(1), 85–96. https://doi.org/10.1080/10615809408248395.

Facoetti, A., & Turatto, M. (2000). Asymmetrical visual fields distribution of attention in dyslexic children: A neuropsychological study. *Neuroscience Letters, 290*(3), 216–218.

Gardner, H. (1999). *Intelligence reframed: Multiple intelligences for the 21st century*. New York: Basic Books.

Greenham, S. L. (1999). Learning disabilities and psychosocial adjustment: A critical review. *Child Neuropsychology, 5*(3), 171–196. https://doi.org/10.1076/chin.5.3.171.7335.

Grills-Taquechel, A. E., Fletcher, J. M., Vaughn, S. R., & Stuebing, K. K. (2012). Anxiety and reading difficulties in early elementary school: Evidence for unidirectional- or bi-directional relations? *Child Psychiatry and Human Development, 43*(1), 35–47. https://doi.org/10.1007/s10578-011-0246-1.

Gross-Tsur, et al. (1995). Developmental right-hemisphere syndrome: Clinical spectrum of the nonverbal learning disability. *Journal of Learning Disabilities, 28*(2), 80.

Ialongo, N., Edelsohn, G., Werthamer-Larsson, L., Crockett, L., & Kellam, S. (1995). The significance of self-reported anxious symptoms in first grade children: Prediction to anxious symptoms and adaptive functioning in fifth grade. *Journal of Child Psychology and Psychiatry, and Allied Disciplines, 36*(3), 427–437. https://doi.org/10.1111/j.1469-7610.1995.tb01300.x.

Kibby, M. Y., Lee, S. E., & Dyer, S. M. (2014). Reading performance is predicted by more than phonological processing. *Frontiers in Psychology, 5*, 960. https://doi.org/10.3389/fpsyg.2014.00960.

Levine, M. (2002). *Educational care*. Cambridge, MA: Educators Publishing Service.

Little, S. S. (1999). The misunderstood child: The child with a nonverbal learning disorder. *Journal of the Society of Pediatric Nurses: JSPN, 4*(3), 113–121. quiz 123-4.

Mahe, G., Doignon-Camus, N., Dufour, A., & Bonnefond, A. (2014). Conflict control processing in adults with developmental dyslexia: An event related potentials study. *Clinical Neurophysiology, 125*(1), 69–76. https://doi.org/10.1016/j.clinph.2013.06.005.

Margari, L., Buttiglione, M., Craig, F., Cristella, A., de Giambattista, C., Matera, E., et al. (2013). Neuropsychopathological comorbidities in learning disorders. *BMC Neurology, 13*(1), 198. https://doi.org/10.1186/1471-2377-13-198.

Margolis, A. E., Pagliaccio, D., Davis, K. S., Thomas, L., Banker, S. M., Cyr, M., et al. (2019). Neural correlates of cognitive control deficits in children with reading disorder. *Brain Imaging and Behavior*. https://doi.org/10.1007/s11682-019-00083-x.

Martin, M. (2007). *Helping children with learning disabilities to flourish*. London: Kingsley.

Mehrabian, A. (1971). *Silent Messages*. Belmont, CA: Wadsworth.

Nowicki, S., & Duke, M. (1992). *Helping the child who doesn't fit in*. Atlanta, GA: Peachtree Publishers.

Ozonoff, S., Rogers, S. J., & Hendren, R. L. (Eds.). (2003). *Autism spectrum disorders: A research review for practitioners*. Washington, DC: American Psychiatric Publishing, Inc..

Palombo, J. (2006). *Nonverbal learning disabilities: A clinical perspective*. New York: WW Norton.

Peck, M. (1985). *Youth suicide*. New York: Springer.

Purvis, K. L., & Tannock, R. (2000). Phonological processing, not inhibitory control, differentiates ADHD and reading disability. *Journal of the American Academy of Child and Adolescent Psychiatry, 39*(4), 485–494. https://doi.org/10.1097/00004583-200004000-00018.

Qin, S., Young, C. B., Duan, X., Chen, T., Supekar, K., & Menon, V. (2014). Amygdala subregional structure and intrinsic functional connectivity predicts individual differences in anxiety during early childhood. *Biological Psychiatry, 75*(11), 892–900. https://doi.org/10.1016/j.biopsych.2013.10.006.

Rourke, B. P. (1988). The syndrome of nonverbal learning disabilities: Developmental manifestations in neurological disease and dysfunction. *The Clinical Neuropsychologist, 4*, 293–330.

Rourke, B. P. (1995). The NLD syndrome and the white matter model. In B. P. Rourke (Ed.), *Syndrome of nonverbal learning disabilities: Neurodevelopmental manifestations* (pp. 1–27). New York: Guilford Press.

Rourke, B. P. (2000). Nonverbal learning disabilities. In A. Klin, F. R. Volkmar, & S. S. Sparrow (Eds.), *Asperger Syndrome*. New York: The Guilford Press.

Rourke, B. P., Young, G. C., & Leenaars, A. A. (1989). A childhood learning disability that predisposes those afflicted to adolescent and adult depression and suicide risk. *Journal of Learning Disabilities*, 22(3), 169–175.

Semrud-Clikeman, M., Fine, J. G., & Bledsoe, J. (2010). Meta-analysis of empirical literature on NVLD. Paper presented at the International Neuropsychological Society.

Semrud-Clikeman, M., Walkowiak, J., Wilkinson, A., & Minne, E. P. (2010). Direct and indirect measures of social perception, behavior, and emotional functioning in children with Asperger's disorder, nonverbal learning disability, or ADHD. *Journal of Abnormal Child Psychology, 38*, 509–519.

Semrud-Clikeman, M., Walkowiak, J., Wilkinson, A., & Gina, C. (2010). Neuropsychological differences among children with Asperger syndrome, nonverbal learning disabilities, attention deficit disorder, and controls. *Developmental Neuropsychology, 35*(5), 582–600.

Ternes, J., Woody, R., & Livingston, R. (1987). A child with right hemisphere deficit syndrome responsive to carbamazepine treatment. *Journal of the American Academy of Child and Adolescent Psychiatry, 26*(4), 586–588. https://doi.org/10.1097/00004583-198707000-00023.

Thompson, S. (1997). *The source for nonverbal learning disorders*. East Moline, IL: Linguisystems.

Varvara, P., Varuzza, C., Sorrentino, A. C., Vicari, S., & Menghini, D. (2014). Executive functions in developmental dyslexia. *Frontiers in Human Neuroscience, 8*, 120. https://doi.org/10.3389/fnhum.2014.00120.

Voeller, K. (1995). Clinical neurological aspects of the right hemisphere deficit syndrome. *Journal of Child Neurology, 10*, 16–22.

Willcutt, E. G., Pennington, B. F., Boada, R., Ogline, J. S., Tunick, R. A., Chhabildas, N. A., et al. (2001). A comparison of the cognitive deficits in reading disability and attention-deficit/hyperactivity disorder. *Journal of Abnormal Psychology, 110*(1), 157–172.

Willcutt, E. G., Pennington, B. F., Olson, R. K., Chhabildas, N., & Hulslander, J. (2005). Neuropsychological analyses of comorbidity between reading disability and attention deficit hyperactivity disorder: In search of the common deficit. *Developmental Neuropsychology, 27*(1), 35–78.

Chapter 9
Working with a Consistent Psychological Theory

It is critical that all of the professionals on the team must be well versed in understanding and dealing with the potential underlying psychological issues presented when someone has NVLD, and they should work from a shared theoretical orientation. An individual with NVLD may often feel confused and anxious about how to respond in social situations. Problems and misunderstandings may frequently occur when attempting to relate to others as a result of deficits in reading social cues, perspective-taking, and literal interpretations, for example. As a child with NVLD matures, they usually have limited free time as they may have to meet with an occupational therapist, psychotherapist, and/or educational specialist in and out of school, and this limits their choices for other after-school activities. The child's parents may make more decisions for him/her sometimes in an effort to protect the child. Their social opportunities are commonly limited or marked with experiences of rejection.

A child with a learning disability, in general, typically experiences limited control and mastery in their life that contributes to an inadequate sense of self (Palombo, 2001). These types of experiences can give rise to unconscious convictions that, as a child, you are at fault for the problems that arise. The child's irrational self-blame and unconscious guilt stem from the responsibility they assume for anything bad that happens to them or significant others. These beliefs are powerful. For example, a child with NVLD who is kept close to the family may incorrectly believe that his parents want him to remain dependent upon them. The family's actual motivation might be to protect them from potential problems. This misunderstanding might cause the child to inhibit desires to be strong and independent because they might have incorrectly assumed that they would displease their parents if they followed this desire (Broitman, 2002).

We find that Weiss' (1993) control mastery theory (CMT) is a way to help families understand the dynamics that go on among the child, the family, the school, and outside therapists and tutors providing support (the helpers). In particular, when the dynamics among the family are challenging, and members of the team are feeling

J. Broitman et al., *NVLD and Developmental Visual-Spatial Disorder in Children*, https://doi.org/10.1007/978-3-030-56108-6_9

particularly discouraged, this theory can shed light on why. A therapist adopting a CMT approach would address these issues by establishing a safe and accepting environment, fostering the child's understanding of themselves and others and how their mind works, and helping them to experience mastery over pathogenic beliefs and gain control in their life. The therapist would encourage a cooperative working relationship between the therapist and the child to disconfirm these pathogenic beliefs. The therapist would believe that the child is highly motivated to disconfirm these beliefs in order to recover the capacity to pursue life goals. This theory is particularly well suited for conceptualizing when there are complicated dynamics between a child with NVLD and their family, peers, and/or school staff. Family members, for example, may feel discouraged and confused because their interpersonal exchanges are chronically static or conflictual.

Weiss would suggest we see this kind of difficult and troubling set of interactions as a part of a child's "testing process" which will be explained in greater detail below. He believed that we all test each other to develop and refine our beliefs throughout life. We do this with our parents, teachers, tutors, siblings, therapists, and friends. Understanding that the feelings we as parents or helpers experience when relating to our children are in part communications from the child can be extremely helpful. These feelings, although often difficult to endure, can offer us direct access to the child's inner world. Parents who can conceptualize the dynamic of the interaction as a "test" or message or communication can better endure and remain sensitive to their child's needs and respond in a way that promotes feelings of emotional safety.

Weiss' theory emphasizes all children's need to adapt to their surroundings. One of the best strategies for doing this is to get along with their parents. Therefore, they are motivated to maintain ties to their parents. This is the attachment part of the theory. They need their parents for survival, safety, love, and security. In order to maintain these ties, a child works to learn as much as possible about their parents. The child infers the moral and ethical principles, which govern their parents' lives, which the parents practice in relation to the child and which the parents expect the child to practice in relation to them. A child struggles to know their parents' whims, needs, and desires. They examine their parents closely in order to sort out what the parents want, expect, and will allow. The child with NVLD, due to their processing difficulties, often has a great deal of trouble sorting this out. It is a difficult task for any child, but when the child experiences difficulties reading interpersonal signals and decoding relationships, and/or their pragmatic language skills are impaired, this can be a truly daunting task!

The child's interpersonal experiences, observations, and inferences are the basis of the conscious and unconscious beliefs that they use to guide them in daily activities. These give rise to beliefs and convictions about how one must behave. Some of these beliefs are maladaptive and significantly constrict the child's ability to develop and function successfully in the world. Weiss refers to these as "pathogenic beliefs" as they are irrational and/or illogical explanations about how one's behavior may have created the difficulty. The child's irrational self-blame and unconscious guilt stem from the responsibility they assume for anything bad that happens to them or their family. These beliefs are powerful. They compel one to behave in certain ways or prohibit certain kinds of behavior. These beliefs warn the child that if they attempt to exercise certain essential functions, or reach certain essential goals, they may put themself in some kind of danger and so risk feeling fear, shame, guilt, loss, or remorse. As these beliefs are overgeneralized, not only to the setting in which the problems occurred but also to the world at large, they can significantly influence the child's future personality development. The child with NVLD's tendency toward misunderstanding signals, and being concrete and literal in their thinking, contributes to this problem.

Pathogenic beliefs stem from a number of sources including identification with a parent's belief or behavior or in compliance with a parent's interpretation of reality. They are created in the misunderstandings that children with NVLD experience on a daily basis. The kind of beliefs a child develops depends on the nature of their specific motivations at the time the beliefs were created and on how the child believes their parents, teachers, and peers reacted to their motivations. The child's beliefs may often be incorrect and exaggerated, or they may be accurate assessments and perceptions of the situation. We therefore believe (and tell all team members and providers) that children come into therapy/school/or tutoring sessions with a plan to overcome their problems, and they test the therapist in predictable ways during therapy. It isn't usually a conscious or fixed plan, but it is more commonly a tentative, flexible strategy for achieving one's goals. It is modified and revised as the therapy progresses. In fact, the child will often mold his plan to the therapist's (tutors, teachers) style, stance, or orientation. The child with NVLD can enter with a variety of irrational beliefs and misunderstandings about themself that lead to the development of social and emotional problems. It is important for professionals and parents to understand the world from within the patient's perspective so that interventions can be helpful! Their symptoms such as compulsions or inhibitions can now also be understood as efforts to avoid dangers foretold by the pathogenic beliefs.

9.1 How Do You Pass a Test?

A test is an unconsciously (sometimes consciously) planned patient behavior that attempts to solicit information about the therapist's/tutor's willingness and ability to help the patient carry out their plan for therapy. Tests vary in how discrete and noticeable they are. The testing behavior may just provide an opportunity for the therapist to intervene in a helpful way, or it may exert a strong demand for the therapist to respond to what the patient is doing or saying. Some tests are barely distinguishable from the patient's normal behavior. Some are obvious. Some occur repeatedly or continuously throughout the therapy. Tests can be passed or failed to varying degrees depending on the therapist's or tutor's responses. Testing is critical, and it cannot be avoided as it is the primary way in which patients attempt to establish if conditions of safety occur with the therapist or tutor to master their childhood traumas, disconfirm their pathogenic beliefs, overcome their pathogenic compliances and identifications, acquire psychological strengths that they lack, and solicit their therapist's/tutor's help in pursuing their therapeutic goals.

Control mastery theory research has identified that there are primarily two kinds of tests (which can co-occur): transference tests (pulling for the therapist or tutor to treat them in the uncomfortable way they experience their parent) and tests by turning passive into active (where the patient takes the role of the traumatizing parent or teacher) (Broitman, 2002). These tests are a way for patients to reevaluate the reality basis for the dangers predicted by the irrational beliefs. It is also often the therapist's best way to understand their patient's emotional experience through understanding the feelings that are being generated in them. In testing, a patient acts in accordance with their belief. Children test in order to find out if the conditions of safety currently exist for making their beliefs conscious. For example, if a child thinks that their parents appear overly worried, they may assume that they must have done something wrong that caused them to worry. Children with NVLD frequently have trouble reading social cues, understanding prosody, and recognizing emotions which will exacerbate this problem. They will, as we all tend to, overgeneralize this experience to believe that they are in fact a worrisome child. To test their belief, they will act particularly worrisome with the therapist or tutor. They hope that the therapist or tutor will not be worried. The professional's calm acceptance and reactions to the child will help them to disconfirm their belief that they (as a worrisome child) caused their parents to worry. If the therapist responds differently than his parents, the child will begin to disconfirm their belief that they were the cause.

9.2 What Happens When You Pass a Test?

Over time, with continued testing and successful responses from the therapist, the child will begin to feel safe and more likely remember significant events and work more productively. This will allow the child to become much more aware of their beliefs and whatever impulses, attitudes, goals, or feelings they have repressed in obedience to these beliefs. Typically, they don't want to face core issues until they are reassured that it will be safe to do so. For example, a child who was impaired by the belief they deserved to be blamed and ridiculed may not remember being blamed until they assure themselves that the therapist will not blame or criticize them in the same manner that their teacher did (Broitman, 2002).

In addition to testing, children also work in treatment by making use of the therapist's interpretations or the tutor's coaching to become more conscious of their beliefs and to realize that they are false and not helpful. This increases the child's control over the effects of their beliefs. They may then become less constrained by the beliefs and less vulnerable to the kinds of trauma to which they were exposed by the beliefs.

Thus, Weiss' theory emphasizes the cooperative working relationship between therapist/tutor and patient to disconfirm their pathogenic beliefs. The child is highly motivated to disconfirm these beliefs in order to recover the capacity to pursue life goals. This theoretical orientation is applicable to all types of treatments and patients in therapy or with a tutor. The way a therapist deals with any type of patient is case specific, meaning it is crucial to consider the specific needs of the person you are dealing with at a particular time. It depends on the particular beliefs that the patient has developed, on which belief the patient is working on at a particular time and the patient's particular way of working. Because this is a case-specific theory, it is particularly well suited for children with NVLD and their families. It requires you to look at how a child is interacting within his or her environment. What are the issues and beliefs that they are developing about themself based on their processing difficulty, and how are these beliefs affecting their entire development?

9.3 Summary

When treating a child with NVLD, all of the team members need to be "therapists" – even when one person is designated to work specifically on the interpersonal or social skills realm. We must share a common psychological understanding regarding a child's conscious and unconscious plan to develop. The team must have regular contact and share information after each session. We often use email summaries to pass among us, so releases of information and permission to use email must be obtained from all participants. We also talk regularly with the LD specialist at the school and individual teachers as needed. If there is another therapist meeting weekly with the child, we suggest the coordinator confer with him/her and the child weekly. In that case, you are the coach, in the role of the child's consultant, there to help him or her get what they need. It is important that the patient is invited and welcomed to contact us with any requests as needed.

We can't emphasize enough how critical it is that all team members must have a shared psychological mindset when working with our patients. The role of and need for therapeutic understanding must be seen, valued, and addressed in every activity and tutoring session. Regular consultation/team meetings can help clarify how aligned your team is. Shared professional training and case presentations will be beneficial. Your team can share readings and theoretical perspectives to find common themes. Programs such as the Brooklyn Learning Center's Homework Therapy understand and address this by having all of their tutoring/coaching done by trained therapists. We suggest you attempt to only work with like-minded professionals who understand and practice with methods that are verbally moderated.

Next in Chap. 10, we offer a step-by-step guide to address the specific challenges the patient is experiencing within the context of the patient's developmental stage.

References

Broitman, J. (2002). *Using control mastery theory to treat the child with NVLD. Symposium on NVLD*. Berkeley, CA: NLDA.

Palombo. (2001). *Learning disorders and disorders of the self in children and adolescents*. New York: Norton and Company.

Weiss, J. (1993). *How psychotherapy works: Process and technique*. New York: Guilford Press.

Chapter 10
Creating a Treatment Plan and Team

A treatment plan and team will need to be created to address the specific challenges the patient is experiencing within the context of the patient's developmental stage. It is critical to address the co-occurring or secondary psychological issues in each of these areas of concern. There will need to be a person designated as the case manager. This can be a psychologist, a parent, or another clinician. This person would be responsible for keeping all members of the team informed about relevant shifts in the situation (e.g., with the family or at school).

The frequency of meetings and contacts will vary with each situation and will be likely to shift as issues arise and are resolved. We begin with more frequent contact and then may reduce the contact when all the necessary team members are on board, and a successful treatment plan is produced and flowing smoothly. In our recommended approach to a treatment team, we suggest sharing information through a central email or chat (being mindful of using secure systems and obtaining written consent to share information from the patient's parent or guardian). Members of the team use the shared chat to provide a weekly report with a brief summary of sessions and offer any information that might be of help to the team.

Texting is often utilized to give each other a heads up regarding an upcoming event, particularly when information is time sensitive and cannot wait for a preplanned or regularly scheduled appointment. Flexibility and availability in real time as issues erupt have proven time and again to be a cornerstone of our success when treating an individual with NVLD. The team leader will be in contact with the pediatrician, school, all of the patient's teachers, and the learning specialist at the school. We would request that school personnel would post assignments, projects, dates of exams, etc. online or through email allowing access to all team members. There should be no surprises for the team with regard to school work requirements. When necessary, assignments should be shortened or adapted, and arrangement for how to do this should be clarified. Homework assignments should be able to be emailed back into school whenever possible. Textbooks should be kept both at home and

J. Broitman et al., *NVLD and Developmental Visual-Spatial Disorder in Children*, https://doi.org/10.1007/978-3-030-56108-6_10

school rather than moved back and forth. The cooperation of the school will be critical, and therefore placement in an appropriate school setting should be carefully considered.

10.1 Choosing the Best Learning Environment

We want to share some of the most important principles to consider and discuss with the family. It is critical that we actively intervene to maximize school success for the child with NVLD. We stress with the family the importance of finding a school environment that reduces the child with NVLD's chances of shame, confusion, and sensory overstimulation. Evaluating the availability of services, including social skills training and alternative learning opportunities, is important as well. Collaboration is also key: a school comfortable with a team approach is required given the often many types of interventions students with NVLD require.

We believe that it is crucial to set up a learning environment that will play to the child's strengths. For example, it may be necessary for professionals to pay attention to the potential impact of physical layout, lights and sounds, crowds, schedules and predictability, classroom size, and numbers of teachers and/or aides when helping a family choose and/or prepare for a school. Teacher substitutions should be infrequent, and classes with shared teaching should be avoided if possible, as continuity and routine offer the best chance for success. The student's schedule needs to be as predictable as possible. They should be prepared in advance for changes in routine, such as assemblies and field trips. These preferences are usually more frequently and easily found in elementary school where there is generally more structure. In middle school, however, it is common to have too many changes and multiple teachers to easily create a safe structure for the student with NVLD.

It is critical that the school personnel understand that students with NVLD will need particular help in interpreting social cues during unstructured periods such during circle time, lunch, or recess. Children with NVLD should not be left unsupervised (especially at lunch or at recess) as they are often the targets for teasing and bullying (Tanguay, 2001, 2002), and these social opportunities provide an opportunity for success if there is appropriate support. Since students with NVLD frequently struggle with transfer and generalization of new skills to different contexts, any plan for success must include a staff that is open to thinking about how this can be accomplished and how to evaluate whether or not it has been successful. Teachers should be encouraged to avoid using figurative speech, or irony, and they should make sure that instruction starts at the concrete level and moves slowly to the more abstract.

When possible, the school should attempt to reduce the number of transitions for the student, such as fewer trips to the locker, fewer classroom changes, etc. as well as help to open their lockers and change quickly for gym. Books and supplies should be arranged such that there will be no need to go back and forth to get items. They should also provide a map of the school and guidance getting to specialists and arranging a buddy system. The school should allow for a mechanism to make careful pickup and drop-off arrangements in order to avoid anxiety and confusion.

Preferential seating should be allowed, and when possible students should sit near and facing the teacher/front row, not close to behaviorally challenged children or children who are noisy or fidgety. Because the learning styles of students with NVLD are concrete and literal, they will be helped by having very specific directions and using rubrics (scoring criteria). These can be very effective as they plot the direction that needs to be taken specifically guiding the learner to broader skill development in a very concrete specific fashion. It's also helpful to front-load expectations, remind children of context, and review their prior knowledge. Multistep tasks will frequently need to be broken into component parts (Tanguay, 2002). Multitasking can prove additional stress and should not be required. Additional time is useful during any transitions, and ample warnings prior to requiring a shift in attention are helpful.

Teachers should be willing to have less visual distraction on walls/boards. Outlines and, for some, graphic organizers can help organize written work because students with NVLD are uni-modal learners. They should not be required to listen and write at the same time. Classroom notes should be emailed home in advance when possible, especially providing notes ahead of lectures in the upper grades. Provide handouts, notes, and outlines for the student instead of requiring copying from the board. When the blackboard is used, use a consistent visual spatial format for organizing information on the blackboard. Write homework assignments in the same area each night. Pre-teaching and reviewing instructional content are also suggested, with the warning to be cautious and make sure that generalization has taken place. Formal cooperative learning can be successful, however, only if care is taken in arranging the makeup of the groups and best with only one consistent teacher (Molenaar-Klumper, 2002).

Because of difficulty in visual tracking, teachers should be open to reducing information on a page and use a flip chart to separate concepts when needed. When assessing the student, teachers should agree to stress content and accuracy in presentations rather than spending too much time on visual appearance. They should allow the student ample opportunities to present information verbally through oral presentations as long as the student is comfortable with this. Because the student may tend to lose their place during a test, it is useful if the school/teacher allows the student to write answers directly on the test sheet rather than requiring them to use a separate answer sheet. Teachers should be aware of the difficulty associated with visual tasks such as matching. Teachers should create simplified test answer sheet layouts and the arrangement of visual–spatial math assignments (no credit should be lost for a correct answer placed in the wrong column or space). Whenever possible, use of graph paper is recommended to keep columns aligned in written math assignments. They should allow the use of a calculator for math-related activities.

Both public and private schools can be options for the child with NVLD, depending on the level of cooperation and what accommodations or modifications are allowed. The public school system will use the Individuals with Disabilities Education Act (IDEA) and create an Individual Education Plan (IEP). The

Individualized Education Program (IEP) is an individualized plan that establishes the educational goals for eligible students for one school year, created at an IEP meeting. However, because NVLD is not a recognized diagnosis, the child's classification for special education services will have to be based on some other diagnosis.

The public school system may then meet a child with NVLD's needs with additional support services; special education in school can be delivered via full inclusion, resource services, or special day classes depending on the individual needs of the child. Services can include speech and language intervention, occupational therapy, etc. Sometimes charter schools might be an option as they often have a simpler physical layout, smaller classes, less disruptive populations, and a higher continuity of students and staff (Table 10.1).

Some private schools may also work, especially those like Mary McDowell School (https://new.marymcdowell.org) in Brooklyn, NY; Winston Preparatory (https://www.winstonprep.edu) in NY, Connecticut, and California; and The Winchendon School (https://winchendon.org) in Brooklyn and Massachusetts. These schools have a focus on teaching children with learning differences using a neuropsychological lens to understand student's struggles based on decades of research on learning and cognition. However, they will not be an option for all children with NVLD due to financial constraints and admissions processes. Other private schools may not be able to provide services and accommodations that would be sufficient for children with NVLD.

Table 10.1 IEP support services

All public schools must provide IEP support
Services available
Integrated Co-Teaching Class (ICT)
Speech therapy (ST)
Occupational therapy (OT)
Transportation
Assistive technology (AT)
Push-in service
Pull-out service
Classroom accommodations
Testing accommodations
Paraprofessional (crisis, health, bus para)
Bilingual services
FM unit
Scribe
Special Education Teacher Support Services (SETSS)
Adaptive Physical Education (APE)
Physical therapy (PT)

There might be an option to take specific problematic subjects (frequently the math and sciences) outside of the school environment through an accredited free-standing specialized program (see, e.g., Northern California's Tilden Academy https://www.tildenprep.com or Fusion https://www.fusionacademy.com) to allow individualized attention. It is imperative to check that any program currently has qualified mental health and special education experts on staff to help with programming and teaching. Some of these programs offer WASC-accredited, college preparatory school for grades 6–12 with approved courses one-on-one and in small groups. With a completely personalized education experience, schedules can be customized, based on availability, for time of day or year that works best for your student and family. They usually use mastery learning, teaching students to 80% (B) or higher level of mastery before moving forward. This allows them to individualize the pace and teaching method to address our children with NVLD's specific range of learning needs, working with students to maximize both their learning and their self-confidence.

In this environment, teachers are able to mentor students in their most challenging subjects, to help them reach their social, emotional, and academic goals, while still having a mainstream school experience. It is, of course, critical to be sure that the particular teachers assigned to our children have been trained in how to best teach children with NVLD. Virtual online classes such as Winston preps's (https://www.winstonprep.edu/distance-learning-program/) are also potentially available for our children with NVLD. WPS's states that their mission is at the core of every decision and plan in their Distance Learning Program which attempts to facilitate the independence and meaningful participation of students with specific learning disabilities through a continuous feedback process that develops skill acquisition and the qualities of sustainable and independent learners. We have found significant success utilizing a combination approach for the most challenging subjects of science and math.

In summary, we stress the importance of finding a school environment that will maximize our students' overall success. We are looking for a school that is open-minded, flexible, and willing to consider the specific unique needs of the *whole* child, not just their disability and remediation needs, recognizing, supporting, and enhancing their strengths as well as their challenges. We close with a description of the key elements (paraphrasing Martin, 2007), for an *ideal* school:

It would have a small building with a simple logical layout; if that was not possible then the ability to limit the child's classes to one section of the school. Any numbering systems such as for classrooms would need to be clear and logical. Classes would occur in one or few classrooms with few doors. There would be a limited number of places to find one's things (lockers, cubbies, desks, closets) near to each other. It would have a low stimulation environment with few distractions. There would be a limited number of teachers, preferably for long periods of time. It would have small structured classes with a consistent schedule and pre-teach the locations of any room changes and use a block schedule. The school would allow extra time for class changes. The staff would be trained in understanding the needs of children with NVLD and willing to assist children with difficult academic subjects *through verbal explanations. In general it has a safe, tolerant, consistent environment that minimizes competition and has no tolerance for bullying. There are supervised, structured social experiences and the teachers are willing and able to provide help deciphering rules. There is wide availability of speech therapy for semantic language and multiple opportunities for children to participate in speech-rich activities such as theater and foreign languages (*Martin, 2007) *p.142).*

10.2 Creating an Action Plan

After the initial clinical interview and reading of test materials, an action plan will need to be developed which considers the patient's age, family's resources, the child's passions, and the areas presenting the most challenge. This will shift as the child grows and develops and as their workload increases. We can't treat all of the child's issues at the same time so the most pressing should be identified, and this should be reevaluated (and adjusted) every 3 months or as is necessary. It's important to leave time and resources for the things they are good at as well as the issues to address. The areas to cover include academic issues which frequently include math and science and paper writing and executive function issues which often impact all subjects and need to be addressed. We have frequently found that our children do not actually learn math or science within the classroom and so have to frequently arrange with an outside service to take over either tutoring the child with NVLD or the entire class by utilizing an individualized personal one-on-one class.

Self-esteem issues are vital especially as related to peer relations and social issues. We have found that they can be best dealt with in individual sessions rather than social skill groups that are often overstimulating and confusing without the possibility of real-time clarifications. We've had a lot of success with sessions involving the use of TV/videos or movies that exaggerate social situations such as sitcoms (e.g., *3rd Rock from the Sun* and *The Big Bang Theory*) or soap operas. Our patients' motor issues have responded to having a personal trainer. Their issues with executive functions are paramount and need constant coaching, attention, scaffolding, and reminders to break things down into individual tasks working toward creating habits and better practices.

We now list the components of a treatment team for a child with NVLD at various times, offered in the order they might be included:

Professional Services:
Developmental pediatrician
Occupational therapist
Physical therapist
Speech and language therapist
Neuropsychologist/psychologist for assessment
Psychotherapist
Child psychiatrist
Social skills specialist
Coach

Educational Intervention and Placement:
Educational therapist
Math tutor
Written expression tutor
Reading comprehension tutor
Educational consultant
Advocate
Specialized school consultant
College counselor
Vocational and rehabilitation consultant
And of course:

Family members:

Child or young adult with NVLD
Parents

Specific information on the role of each of these professionals can be found in *Treating NVLD in Children: Professional Collaborations for Positive Outcomes* (Broitman & Davis, 2013). There you will find each practitioner's methods (as it relates to their field), regarding the treatment of children with NVLD, including the instruments of assessment used to assess the area(s) of difficulty, examples of a treatment plan, illustrating how they might work with a child with NVLD, and sample school or parent reports for their discipline with typical recommendations/referrals for other professional services. We go on in Chap. 11 to discuss how to help your patients' families best support their child with NVLD's psychological growth and development.

References

Broitman, J., & Davis, J. M. (2013). *Treating NVLD in children: Professional collaborations for positive outcomes*. New York: Springer.

Martin, M. (2007). *Helping children with nonverbal learning disabilities to flourish*. London: Jessica Kingsley.

Molenaar-Klumper, M. (2002). *Non- verbal learning disabilities: Characteristics, diagnosis and treating within an educational setting*. London: Jessica Kingsley, Publishers.

Tanguay, P. B. (2001). *Nonverbal learning disabilities at home*. London: Jessica Kingsley, Publishers.

Tanguay, P. B. (2002). *Nonverbal learning disabilities at school*. London: Jessica Kingsley, Publishers.

Chapter 11
Working with Your Patient's Family

We work very closely with our patient's parents or partners and spouse to help them deal with the very common difficult feelings and experiences such as anxiety, fragility, frustration, and confusion. Family members often alternate between being too worried and guilty, or feelings of anger, irritation, avoidance, denial, or loss of patience. Confused, feeling overwhelmed, or simply tired, they often react with frustration. Parents can feel guilty believing that they have damaged their child because they haven't been steady or done the right things. This dynamic can lead to guilt, confusion, anxiety, worry, and demoralization on everyone's part. Since children cannot understand their parent's reactions, they often end up feeling overly responsible for their parent's behavior and then blame themselves. They often believe the distress the parent feels is their fault and the child can feel a variety of troubling emotions such as depressed, anxious, stupid, crazy, and confused. These difficult feelings can cause additional problems for everyone. With help in understanding this process, parents and professionals can prevent or minimize this from happening.

Parents can be taught how to deal with their own frustrations, understand their limitations, and realize that their own family histories and dynamics will influence the expectation they have for their children. Parents can be shown the additional complicated impact these expectations will have on children with NVLD. Making the link between parental frustration and the message it gives their child can be very useful.

Many individuals with NVLD have learned how to compensate for their disability by verbally persuading others (teachers, parents, counselors, siblings, etc.) to intervene for them when tasks or situations become too difficult (Foss 1991). Matte and Bolaski (1998) address the concern that complying with such requests might be a disservice and promotes incompetence. We find that this is often a question for parents, frequently asking what is helping vs. holding their child back from learning to do it on their own. We are not in favor of it, but suggestions of a "tough love" approach are often cited as well. We, however, believe that the practitioner must

J. Broitman et al., *NVLD and Developmental Visual-Spatial Disorder in Children*, https://doi.org/10.1007/978-3-030-56108-6_11

monitor, balance, and/or titrate the level of frustration being experienced by the child so that they are encouraged to increase their social skills repertoire but without becoming hopeless and disaffected. It is a therapeutic balancing act. We find we have the most success follows first providing adequate training and support.

Rourke (1995) acknowledges the difficult tension between protecting the vulnerable child with NVLD from failure while simultaneously trying to expand their horizons. In Matte and Bolaski's (1998) clinical experience, they say they have also found that honesty, clarity, and directness are essential in the child developing self-worth and self-awareness and in fostering an understanding and acceptance of ability rather than fostering overemphasis of disability. Rourke (1995) stressed that it is necessary to cultivate realistic expectations for the person with NVLD, taking account of both assets and deficits. Foss (1991) and Matte and Bolaski's (1998) concur, and we suggest creating scaffolding from which the child can begin to develop skills. We believe that the key is *working with* the child to help them to increase their capacity for independent activity. Whitney (2000) also suggests that clinicians need to bridge the gaps for their NVLD clients until they can develop the needed skills for themselves. We believe that these collaborations will develop competence and self-esteem and work to help parents overcome their fears of holding their children back.

Martin (2007), herself the mother of a child with NVLD, acknowledges the burden parents of children with NVLD have to create a safe home environment. She stresses the importance of providing a psychologically safe refuge free from the exhausting demands of the outside world. Just accomplishing the basic learning activities can be exhausting for these children. They will also have a greater need for parental assistance in all areas of life over the course of their lifespan. Parents will need assistance in managing these tasks without fears of infantilizing their children (Rourke 1995) or making them overly dependent. Professionals can and must help parents recognize the appropriateness of parental intervention and involvement (Whitney 2000).

Professionals should teach parents to understand why their children are vulnerable so that they can advocate for their children. Armed with knowledge, parents can correct the ignorance which often fuel the criticisms leveled at them. Martin (2007) cautions that it takes a great deal of time to act as their mediator to the world but offers the following suggestions to make the time worthwhile: Ask your child with NVLD questions to stretch their thinking. Help them to see patterns – to understand and anticipate routines and schedules. Explicitly explain the use of schedules. Develop an open and non-judgmental relationship which will promote their allowing you to know with what they need help. Regularly check in with them regarding how things are going. Specifically ask about their social interactions and demystify the novelty. Encourage their reflectivity through modeling/verbalizing finding solutions to challenges. Make your home a "psychological" haven for the child (reducing stress and stimulation). Limit the number of new experiences so that they have the ability to practice and master tasks. Accept that homework will take longer and your child will need your assistance and work with the school to best manage assignments for relevance. Keep duplicates of books to avoid the issues related to forgetting to bring them home. Allow them to dictate to you when constructing maps and graphs and diagrams. Practice activities with them before they perform them independently (such as taking the bus) so that they will be successfully able to manage on their own and obtain as much independence and autonomy as they can.

Martin (2007) addresses the need for families to step in and help their child progress in an appropriate developmental fashion, noting that each child will have different skills. Some may never learn to drive, while others can become good drivers with assistance. The life skills required for independent living such as dating and managing social relationships, managing a checkbook, laundry, cooking, and housekeeping will have to be carefully and explicitly taught. Martin goes on to reflect upon the difficulty families have balancing their wishes to promote their child's independence and the realities that require additional interventions. She encourages a progressive approach in which one withdraws support whenever it is no longer needed but is ever ready to put them back in if the child encounters something new and novel and cannot quite figure out how to access and generalize previously learned material.

11.1 Suggestions for Parents and Family Members

What follows are our suggestions for ways to take the above principles and operationalize them so that parents can improve their communications and interactions with their child with NVLD. As a parent, the most important thing you can do for your child with NVLD is to actually listen to them and make them feel that you care about their feelings and perceptions of the situation, even if that does not match your own. Listen to your child and focus on trying to figure out where they are in pain (physical, mental, etc.). You can show you're listening by actively and promptly responding to what they say, even if that's requesting more information or saying you don't understand. You can also show active involvement by repeating back what you think you've understood so that they can correct you. Throughout this active listening, the focus should be on trying to solve those issues with your children as *active participants* – that means finding solutions that actually solve the problem for them rather than what would work for you, or fit a specific diagnosis, or be easiest. If a solution doesn't fit, keep looking. If a solution partially fits, keep looking.

Accept that your child already knows that they are different in some way, whether or not they have received or have been told about an official diagnosis. While your feelings around a diagnosis may involve worries about labels and inevitable limitations, know that for your child, thinking there is "something unknown and wrong with them" is infinitely worse. In fact, *having a diagnosis* means your child is now exposed to the idea that there are other people like them out there, which is much more hopeful than thinking they are literally alone.

Accept that your child's interpretation/perspective is *valid* and the most important issue at stake. You can show this in a variety of ways, including listening properly (see above). You should also verbally emphasize your love and acceptance for your child through explicit and repetitive language and behaviors. Try and remove extra challenges for your child, i.e., take tasks or responsibilities off their plate and do not discuss finances or burdens of potential solutions. By removing these things, you are not "enabling them" or preventing them from developing necessary skills. In fact the opposite is true; you are providing them space to learn and develop at their own pace.

Processing what it means to have a diagnosis and intervention is difficult for the whole family and not just the individual with NVLD. Try not to get caught up in your own feelings, at least in front of them. This process is likely to be at least somewhat painful and guilt-inducing for parents (and at times the siblings), as they come to better understand the challenges and pain the child is going through. The family will have to accept that there is a limited extent to which their pain and guilt can help alleviate their child's pain. Experiment with solutions and ways of thinking in response to your child's needs.

One of the most powerful things you can do to support your child and to prove that you are listening actively to their needs is to advocate for your child – do not put the burden of figuring everything out on them alone. You can do this by helping with finding solutions, including doctors, experts, products, etc. Help with scheduling and research for interventions, therapies, and more. Be actively and verbally interested in how appointments and experiments go. When age-appropriate, actively look for resources/books/blogs written by people with similar/the same issues and pass them on to your children, in order to *actively solicit* their opinions and feedback in order to continuously refine your understanding of their needs. These can be great ways to have conversations about how your child is feeling and to identify methods of further support.

One area of support you can provide for your child is to help develop processes. A lot of where your child's energy gets used up every day is often in attempting to accomplish tasks that you as a neurotypical may find unthinkably easy. Best not to start an intervention with "don't worry, this will be easy." Helping your child identify weak points and then, crucially, build simple and straightforward processes to cope/compensate can help give them confidence and skills going forward (Tsatsanis and Rourke 2003). A therapist/therapy team will often also work on these sorts of skills, especially in academic settings, but the need for processes like this also applies to non-academic settings which are a great way for you to get directly involved, if you and your child want that level of involvement. Tricky areas can include chores: breakdown tasks like "do the dishes" into steps to set boundaries, i.e., how full does the dishwater need to be to run it? Does doing the dishes include putting away leftovers? Does it include wiping down the counter? Do these chores with your child and talk through the steps involved.

Another area where you may be able to help is with specific types of communication, i.e., "essay introductions," "request emails," response to "how are you," or "disclosing your diagnosis." These types of general communication tasks can be broken down into a regular template; talk through and write down these processes with your child. Furthermore, socializing in general is often something your child will want but find overwhelming and have trouble achieving. Having discussions to identify what kind of social situations your child most enjoys (likely 1:1 or small group and around a structured activity) is key and then working with your child to set benchmarks for success, i.e., sit with one friend at least twice per week at lunch, or join one new weekly activity over the next few months, or attend two parties this year, etc.

Finally, help your child identify triggers that cause stress or overstimulation: likely a consistent problem underlying other weak areas is not knowing where your child's boundaries are with socialization, environmental stimulation, etc. Going through each individual area and trying to talk through boundaries enable you and your child to be able to plan in advance what may work versus what may be too much. In Chap. 12 we address the need to learn from our patients how to offer techniques and interventions tailored to their specific needs.

References

Foss, J. (1991). Nonverbal learning disabilities and remedial interventions. *Annual of Dyslexia, 41*, 128–140.

Martin, M. (2007). *Helping children with nonverbal learning disabilities to flourish*. London: Jessica Kingsley.

Matte, R. R., & Bolaski, J. A. (1998). Nonverbal learning disabilities: An overview. *Intervention in School & Clinic, 34*(1), 39–43.

Rourke, B. P. (1995). The NLD syndrome and the white matter model. In B. P. Rourke (Ed.), *Syndrome of nonverbal learning disabilities: Neurodevelopmental manifestations* (pp. 1–27). New York: Guilford Press.

Tsatsanis, K. D., & Rourke, B. P. (2003). Syndrome of nonverbal learning disabilities: Effects on learning. In A. H. Fine & R. A. Kotkin (Eds.), *Therapist's guide to learning and attention disorder* (pp. 109–145). Amsterdam: Academic.

Whitney, R. V. (2000). *The nonverbal learning disorder guide for teachers, parents, employers, and therapists*. Campbell, CA: Lighthouse Project.

Chapter 12
Learning from Our Patients

As we have previously noted, every patient presents differently with different assets and challenges. Therefore, the single best source of information we have about a patient is the patient themselves. However, our patients have not necessarily learned how to articulate their feelings and reactions in an organized and medically rigorous way. Regardless, the information they report is often our most important and accurate source of their challenges.

It is imperative that we make sure that we understand our patient's diagnosis and share that information with them. We must talk to their family members, teachers, and other relevant people as well as keep up to date on the literature and blog posts (especially by those within that specific NVLD community). Your highest priority and responsibility is quite simply to listen to your patient. Since it is easy for people with NVLD to misunderstand communications, it is important to (1) ask them to repeat back to you what they have heard you say and (2) repeat back for them what you are hearing. Make it clear that you are asking continuously and explicitly for correction and clarification to *improve your understanding of their experience*, not to make their experience fit into a preexisting mental model or methods of intervention.

A source of information about treatments and interventions that is often overlooked is the online community of people, including adults, with NVLD (see, e.g., NVLD Project https://nvld.org). Blogs, Facebook groups, etc. are useful sources of information to help find effective techniques for coping with NVLD. These sites also provide narratives of experiences of having NVLD that may resonate for your patient but which they may not yet be able to articulate. See, for example, NLD-In-Common Listserv: NLDAdult, for those with NLD ages 18 and older. Go to http://groups.yahoo.com/group/NLDAdults. NLDCollege: For those with NLD who are enrolled in a college/university program. Go to http://groups.yahoo.com/group/NLDCollege/.

One way of developing communication and articulation around this very tricky topic could be to have your patient read memos/blogs/books/articles written by

J. Broitman et al., *NVLD and Developmental Visual-Spatial Disorder in Children*, https://doi.org/10.1007/978-3-030-56108-6_12

other patients/students with NVLD to highlight what speaks to their experience and then to share them with you and their teachers, friends, and family members. Recognizing themselves in others' experience is both psychologically powerful and therapeutically useful to begin and continue discussions around topics for which patients do not yet have a developed vocabulary. Alternatively, they might write and share their own memos/blogs/books/articles in order to best communicate their thoughts, feelings, and needs.

By the time someone sees an LD specialist for treatment, they may well have already had negative experiences (thus why they have kept searching) with other professionals. Explicitly acknowledging and inviting information about past problems in order to avoid them and give agency to the patient could be a useful technique to separate yourself from previous bad experiences. Likewise, language or techniques that may be appropriate with neurotypical patients/students, for example, validating feelings without problem-solving, focusing on emotional issues before practical ones, or asking open-ended feelings based questions as starting points, may not work. This might be both because there is often a strongly problem-based environmental reason that has brought the patient to an LD specialist as opposed to a more general therapist/tutor and because they may not yet have developed a language to helpfully answer open-ended questions.

The key is to show in both words and consistent behavior that you are open to expressions of emotions, especially negative ones like frustration, anger, fear, etc. The process of getting to an NVLD specialist often involves years of being told to conform in some impossible way, and patients are often aware without understanding that "something is different" and "wrong," and often trained to try and "suck it up" or "fit in," rather than actually express their feelings, reactions, and emotions. This is the year-long social training you will have to patiently try to disrupt.

All of this goes toward the psychological goal of helping patients, even children, feel like active participants in their own treatment, with appropriate amounts of agency, rather than as passive recipients of treatments determined by qualified adult experts. Given that NVLD presentation is quite individualized and changes over time, ensuring patients feel able to actively contribute their feelings, reactions, and ideas to the treatment process is important in directing interventions to areas of highest immediate need, building sustainable skills, and promoting self-awareness and self-confidence.

One concrete way of ensuring this framework of encouraging agency is apparent from the outset is making patients aware of how the team is sharing information about treatments and the patient, to ensure that the feeling of "being talked about behind one's back," whether accurate or not given the difficulties in assessing nonverbal social cues, is avoided. While it is likely not appropriate to include the patient in all those communications, their awareness and permission for such information to be shared, even if a child or minor, is important for engendering feelings of transparency and proactive teamwork toward improving their experience in their environment, rather than feelings of needing to be "fixed" in a more physical/medical sense.

In addition to psychological and academic issues, the importance of environmental factors cannot be overstated. What for neurotypical people may barely register as an environmental stressor is often vividly – too vividly – present for our patients with NVLD. This can mean that what presents immediately as psychological, academic, social, or life skills challenges may in fact have their roots in sensory issues. Sensory issues could be presenting a barrier to understanding or completing a set task/dealing with a particular situation, which may appear to be taking the form of content incomprehension or "bad behavior," may in fact be a response to an unnoticed sensory issue. Sensory sensitivities can include reactions to issues like fabrics, temperature, or light that take energy and concentration to consciously ignore, thus diminishing abilities to "deal with" or focus on more usual tasks. It may also take the form of nonverbal social uncertainties which can be expressed as social anxiety, social awkwardness, etc. It is highly unlikely that social issues signal a lack of desire for social success. Therefore, investigating in detail environmental issues is key to successfully building a sustainable NVLD intervention. See Chap. 13 and the Environmental checklist in the appendix for a detailed discussion of assessing these factors.

Another area that will be particularly important to explore with your patient will be their desires regarding friendships and dating and gender and sexual identity. Some people with NVLD will not want to date, and that needs to be validated as a legitimate preference, while others will actively want to pursue this and may want help with reading body language, understanding nuances such as sarcasm in communication, and managing new relationships. This is likely to be an uncomfortable area of discussion for many patients, and one of the most important recommendations of this chapter and this book overall is to listen to your patient and be consistently clear and supportive about working with their priorities and goals, rather than assumed ones based on normative standards based on age range or academic intelligence.

In terms of working with your patients' parents, this may or may not be part of the discussion around sexuality and dating, but clarity, confidentiality, safety, and support are key to ensure patients feel comfortable discussing this topic. If parents have specific safety reasons for not wanting this topic addressed, those can be discussed, but in general we advise that if a patient is willing and interested in discussing romance, dating, and sexuality, it is healthier for all involved to be open and supportive about these discussions and not make assumptions about the ability of people with NVLD to successfully date and have romantic relationships. In our clinical experience, people with NVLD may have extra difficulties finding romantic relationships due to social challenges but can succeed with the right support and partner, as with other areas.

Understanding what your patients are actually interested in regarding gender and sexuality is important, as with all other aspects of their lives, assuming neurotypical standards, desires, or progressions may in fact hinder true understanding and support. For example, while "typical" high schoolers may be interested in dating, that may not be true for students with NVLD who are more focused on achieving academic clarity and success or who simply are not interested or ready at this "normal" age. Similarly, if someone with NVLD is interested in dating, the methods and progressions that may be "expected" may also not suit, for example, bars are not friendly to someone whose main skills are in verbal conversation rather than non-verbal body language.

Some people with NVLD may want to date and find relationships; however, their idea of a relationship may be different to "standard" expectations, around length of time spent with a partner, what kinds of activities would be fun to do as a date, or around preferences, either behavioral or environmental, around intimacy. Directly discussing these specific aspects, as much as your patient is comfortable, is key to helping them develop specific processes, plans, and skills to attempt dating. Just like with academics or non-romantic social engagement, discussing plans and ideas and breaking these down into concrete and linear steps are the key to success for NVLD brains.

NVLD relationship therapist and coach Benjamin Meyer, MSW (https://nvld.org/dating-success-strategies-nvld/), has a number of dating tips for NVLD people. He mentions the importance of working with social and/or therapeutic networks, mainly friends and peers, to explicitly discuss dating practices, norms, behaviors, and even act out dating scenarios to help people with NVLD get used to interpreting facial expressions and other body language in this specific context.

Moira, reflecting on her experiences, says that: "Dating before my diagnosis was very stressful, as I always felt there was a lot of information I was missing in terms of understanding what I was "supposed" to do, and interpreting my partner's wants and needs as well. I definitely ended up in situations where I did not understand how I had gotten there, and was not sure how to comfortably move forward." Dating and intimacy also raised challenges for Moira's sensory issues, "Kissing for a long time felt too wet, too close, too hot, to be comfortable, much less enjoyable, on a purely sensory level." What proved to be successful, however, for Moira were exactly the kinds of tips outlined on Meyers' website (https://benjaminmeyerlcsw.com/), including engaging with potential dates via dating apps and using her strengths in attention to detail and memory to start conversations around details mentioned in their profiles, rather than generic openers. This allowed her to much more quickly assess compatibility in terms of interests, thus increasing the chances that an in-person date would have at least some known good topics of conversation to work with. Likewise, primarily for sensory reasons, Moira made sure that all her dates were in places and with activities that encouraged long-form communication, to utilize her comfort and skill in her verbal abilities.

Once a relationship is established, it will be important to help your patient think through how one decides when and how or if to self-disclose to a partner. This is an important issue without a correct answer. It will be important to talk together about the pros and cons for your individual patient at each particular time. One of the key factors around this decision is finding a romantic partner with whom the person with NVLD feels comfortable being very honest with, as verbal communication is a core strength of NVLD and lying through omission and body language can be quite difficult, so ensuring patients prioritize communication skills with partners is key.

For Moira, these methods successfully resulted in forming a strong relationship built on open communication. She disclosed her diagnoses as well as specific sensory issues to her boyfriend and was able to have a productive and safe conversation around the relationship and intimacy in mutually beneficial ways. Moira said "for me, the best romantic and friend relationships have always been with people I can be very honest with, not just about my feelings, but also feeling safe and accepted to ask for clarification about their feelings when I am unsure. Having built strong friendships and developed further skills through those processes, I was able to find a great romantic partnership as well."

Next in Chap. 13 we consider the timing of interventions. This chapter will help you navigate how to decide which issues to address, in what order, including how to break down and create a plan for each specific problem your patient faces.

References

Benjamin Meyer, MSW. https://nvld.org/dating-success-strategies-nvld

NLDCollege. *For those with NLD who are enrolled in a college/university program*. Go to http://groups.yahoo.com/group/NLDCollege/

NLD-In-Common Listserv. *NLDAdult: For those with NLD ages 18 and older*. Go to http://groups.yahoo.com/group/NLDAdults

NVLD Project. https://nvld.org

Chapter 13
Choosing What to Work on First in Therapy/Tutoring

Given the possibility of previous negative experiences with a professional, your patient may test you to see if you are going to repeat the difficult interactions and re-traumatize them. Your patient might need to begin their work with you by first getting permission to express emotions, especially negative ones. You might experiment with using different modalities of communication/expression, i.e., in person vs. phone or video (even if geographically near) vs. text vs. email, etc., to determine what provides your patient with the most safety and opportunity to accurately assess the dangers for them in working with you.

It's important that you make sure you respond to your patient within the expected timeframe you have created together. We have found therapist availability has been a big factor in connecting with our patients with NVLD. Frequency of meeting has varied, and allowing for a flexible schedule when possible, is often useful. Text communications allow for real-time interventions as well. It is best to acknowledge their emotions and problems clearly and specifically. General responses such as "I'm sorry you're feeling that way" can come across as platitudes, whereas "I'm sorry you're feeling that way, can you tell me more about the feeling you mentioned?," will seem more responsive. Explore with your patient whether validation or problem-solving is preferred in general or in each specific situation. Use targeted questions to ascertain your patients' feelings/agenda to show legitimate interest rather than adult general platitudes.

13.1 Diagnosing Environmental Challenges

Sensory issues are essentially someone finding touch, sound, light, taste, or other sense-based stimuli either too much or too little in their effect, compared to the range of "normal." These issues can often be unnoticed, including by the affected person, since what is considered normal is subjective, making it hard to understand

J. Broitman et al., *NVLD and Developmental Visual-Spatial Disorder in Children*, https://doi.org/10.1007/978-3-030-56108-6_13

what someone else's range of sensory reactions are in comparison to one's own. However, overreacting to sensory stimuli can have a hugely problematic effect on one's ability to function with the same behaviors as others; sensory stimuli that may be completely unnoticeable to one person are so overwhelming to another that, for example, they cannot follow a conversation. While many sensory tests also check for hypersensitivity to stimuli (feeling more than normal), this is less likely to cause behavioral issues from stimuli overexposure. In many cases, there are low-cost, low-effort ways that sensory issues can be addressed, and testing is mainly a matter of guided self-reflection. Therefore, it is efficient to check for sensory issues as part of a general diagnostic process for anyone potentially being screened for any behavioral issues.

A full list of diagnostic questions to check for sensory processing issues in both children and adults (including adolescents) can be found from places like Sensory-Processing-Disorder.com. The below is an abbreviated list developed by the authors to address sensory issues most commonly seen in our experience with our NVLD patients. In the direct sensory categories, a patient should be asked about and observed about their reactions to light (brightness, inside versus outside, colors of light, screen color/brightness), heat (temperature, humidity, sunburn, wind), sound (total amount of noise, difficulty filtering out background noise, sound sensitivity at different times of day), tactile (shampoo/thick liquids, clothing material/tags, toothbrushing/oral input, hair brushing, amount or proximity of touch, touching "messy" things like sand, glue, etc.), and taste/texture (mushy, spicy, acidic, mixed tastes, mixed textures, mixed colors requiring visual food separation).

Sensitivities in these areas can translate into what is observed as behavioral abnormalities that may have purely or combined sensory causes. For example, difficulty filtering out background noise from the conversation a patient is meant to be participating in could present as ignoring a conversational partner or failing to follow the logic of a discussion, when in fact, the patient is unable to distinguish the words they are meant to be following from other conversations in the vicinity, such as during group discussions in a classroom or a meeting in a coffee shop. Another example would be seemingly inconsistent reactions toward social interactions with others, when in fact the environment suggested for these activities (a sunny playground with a rough playing surface versus a shaded park with soft grass) may be a contributing factor for inconsistent willingness or ability to socialize normally.

Beyond these immediate sensory stimuli, there are other environmental factors to consider, particularly in terms of observed behavioral or social abnormalities. As hinted at above, the physical aspects of an environment may be important, including how crowded an area might be, size, amount of light, amount of noise, temperature level, or clothing requirements. For example, the discomfort of a particular item of mandatory school clothing may in fact be a cause for a child not enjoying school, rather than anything in particular about the school itself. Similerly, someone with a temperature sensitivity may dislike smaller spaces that can heat up quickly from body heat and therefore prefer larger work areas or classrooms. There are also specifically nonverbal aspects of social environments which are likely worth considering, such as the amount of structure the activity provides and how familiar the patient is with how this activity proceeds. Relatedly, understanding the number of known versus unknown people, total number of people a patient may be expected to interact with, and whether there are additional aspects to manage, such as food or alcohol. These factors may combine with logistical aspects of environments such as amount and complexity of transit time, familiarity of transit route, and flexibility of arrival and departure times from the event.

Finally, it is important to understand that sensory issues are often underdiagnosed because of the subjectivity issues noted above but also due to societal pressures. Due to the subjectivity of understanding any individual's sensory perceptions, understanding that one has sensory perceptions that significantly differ from others is usually a realization that takes years to fully develop, much less convince others of. It is not a problem that is often discussed explicitly, even in situations where sensory sensitivities are acute enough for patients and even their families to unconsciously or quietly develop coping mechanisms in response.

Therefore, there is a final category of challenge in that a patient with sensory issues may need assistance developing coping strategies for the psychological aspects of dealing with difficult environments. These issues may precipitate social anxiety and psychological perceptions, sometimes bolstered by outside influences, of how the patient "should" feel and behave in different environments. These are often behavioral expectations learned from reactions about how the patient is expected to react before sensory sensitivities are understood and addressed and often consider long-lasting psychological issues due to repeated training to repress sensory reactions that the patient perceives no one else to be feeling. Sensory sensitivities, therefore, while likely also caused by differences in brain function, must be treated holistically both as an expression of a neurological difference but also with a strong psychological component.

13.2 Treating Environmental and Sensory Issues

There are a wide variety of interventions that can help address sensory and environmental issues, but perhaps more so than in other areas of interventions, the best adaptations, items, and practices for your patient are highly specific to each individual, and some amount of experimentation will likely be needed to find the right combination of methods for the best results. The following describes some examples of interventions for various direct sensory/environmental issues as well as secondary impacts (e.g., for academic work), but these should be considered very much as examples rather than overarching or guaranteed recommendations from the authors.

For most sensitivities, there are essentially two main options in every case: change the environment or find protective/adaptive mechanisms for the individual to use regardless of environment. For light sensitivities, this could include changing the method of lighting rooms – upward facing lights (like standing lamps) with yellow bulbs produce more diffuse light as compared to floor-facing overhead bright white lights. One can purchase different colored bulbs as needed for one's own home. There are four types of light bulbs: incandescent, compact fluorescent (CFL), halogen, and light-emitting diode (LED). Lumens refer to the amount of light that is radiated or the brightness of the bulb. Similar to watts, the higher the lumen, the brighter the light. Light bulbs are available in different colors: candlelight, warm white, neutral white, and daylight. The colors are measured on the Kelvins (K) temperature scale. Colors on the color temperature scale that range from about 2700 K to 3000 K are called warm colors. Sunset and sunrise typically feature light in the warm color temperature range, a bit lower in number (about 1800 K) than the light of a warm incandescent bulb. Moonlight is a bit bluer or cooler, in the 4100 K range. Cool white is often 4000 K, going up to 6000 K or 7000 k – which is a really blue light. Check out Table 13.1 Color temperature chart to see which Kelvin number is best for your individual preferences.

Unfortunately, in many academic and public spaces, overhead extremely bright white lights are utilized. Therefore, we recommend experimenting with tinted glasses. Some patients in our experience have had success with gray and black tinted glasses, essentially traditional sunglasses, but some patients have found more success with dark yellow (2x darker than yellow ski goggles) or other colored lenses. Another aspect to keep in mind when trying on glasses is the feel of the glasses themselves, in terms of the weight of the frames, whether your patient feels comfortable with nose pads, the extent to which the frames are visible to the wearer, etc.

For temperature/humidity/sunburn/clothing/tactile issues, the key will likely be adapting outfits to accommodate layers of different materials and weights of fabric as it is generally harder to change the temperatures/environments a patient is exposed to, and therefore the focus will likely be on creating adaptive strategies. There are also options like sun protective clothing or powder-based sunscreen which could be useful in some situations for patients who do not like the thick feeling of regular sunblock. For heat sensitivities, options like sweat blocking wipes, anti-chafing/sweat creams, removable perspiration pads, etc. can also be effective. Heat issues may also arise when learning skills like cooking, in which case focusing on learning recipes that require minimal long-term interaction with stoves/ovens (i.e., through one-pot, instant-pot, or "throw in the oven and roast") is likely to be a better starting place.

Table 13.1 Color temperature chart

Candlelight (1000 K–2600 K): Light bulbs with less than 2000 K give off a dim glow, similar to candlelight
Warm white (2600 K–3000 K): This is the standard color of incandescent bulbs. They are typically used as ceiling and wall lights
Neutral white (3000 K–5000 K): This cool white-colored option provides a bright light
Daylight (5000 K+): This provides a crisp light that is similar to daylight

For issues with sound, there are a variety of possible interventions, depending on the specific subproblem being addressed. For being overwhelmed with sheer level of noise, foam earplugs used for professional shooters can often be bought in bulk and are more flexible and comfortable than generic earplugs without being much more expensive. They can also be used in more public places than more visible ear protections that may be socially problematic or at night to ensure high-quality sleep. However, over-ear noise protectors or noise-canceling headphones are also a useful option. Bose tends to have good noise-canceling headphones, and there are of course many alternative brands. In terms of adapting to situations where the sound issue is filtering out relevant from background noise, minimizing the frequency with which your patient must endure these environments is likely a positive adaptive strategy. If required to be in these atmospheres, being able to sit with their back against the wall or ideally in a corner is likely going to be the least problematic area, as patients can use visual distinguishers to help differentiate between different conversations. In classrooms, a FM lapel microphone on a teacher can transmit directly to the impacted student eliminating the element of background noise.

For tactile issues, patients with many kinds of sensory issues as well as a range of anxiety issues have found weighted blankets to be soothing, so much so that these products are now widely available through large commercial websites. One thing to note, however, is that these weighted blankets are still relatively light; should your patient want a heavier blanket, specialty autism order sites are likely the better solution than mainstream commercial options. In terms of clothing issues, the guiding rule is likely to be soft and relatively seamless, for which there is an increasing range of options, but may take some experimenting to find particular materials, cuts, or brands that work best for your patient. In addition to fabric type, understanding your patient's preferences in terms of collar (tight, loose, close or far from the neck, etc.), general fit (tight or loose), sleeve length (around the wrists or not), etc. may be particular areas worth focusing on.

For secondary sensory sensitivities, for example, issues around socializing in unpleasant or unfamiliar environments or affecting academic behavior, the most important intervention is going to be psychological and twofold. First, listen to your patient, and try to explicitly understand exactly what environmental impacts your patient is reacting to. Secondly, do your best collectively with the patient and the whole team to collect as much environmental information as possible about new situations or places so that appropriate interventions, adaptations, and psychological planning can be prepared.

13.3 Academics Issues

Carefully review your patient's issues and concerns regarding their academic performance. Help them make adjustments as needed in the amount of things on their workload including how many things are on their plate simultaneously. Talk through looming deadlines to consider frequency in general, turnaround times, and how the deadlines compare across assignments. Review the school's expectations, including their allowance for multiple drafts and getting feedback. Help them with prioritization of importance, knowledge of format, content, and grading expectations. Since the students' executive functions are compromised, help them break down assignments and tasks both in content and scheduling and type of work, i.e., math, science, or written expression.

Address and acknowledge the emotional/traditional psychological work dealing with family relationships, perceptions of priority, and perceptions around the amount of help "deserved" represented by money, attention, timeliness of response, etc. As verbal and reading skills are often a strength, interventions in this area can focus on talking through the creation of processes that can then be written down in lists or bullet points to allow patients to keep track of what has worked and how to tackle new tasks or challenges. Focusing on specificity, especially developed through verbal discussion and then confirmed through written processes, shows tangible experiments and progress to the patient, treatment team, parents, and wider community (i.e., school).

Your patient is also likely to need significant help with life skills training, especially as they mature, and these are likely to be related to sensory issues. Potential priority areas include the following:

1. Cooking: recipe planning/learning, grocery shopping, meal planning, and cooking.
2. Laundry: learning to use machines, buying appropriate cleaning materials, and knowing how to sort/treat laundry.
3. Household maintenance: knowing which cleaning items to buy, knowing how to use and how often to use cleaning items, and basic information on heating, smoke alarms, light bulb switching, etc.
4. Budgeting: is a potentially difficult task for our patients with NVLD. They will need your help to learn how to build a spreadsheet and what to put on the spreadsheet – including how to estimate/level of detail required, how to track spending, how to reasonably adjust spending, and how one balances skills/chores (i.e., cooking, laundry, personal hygiene, etc.) in general and with work/school obligations.
5. The area of dating, sexual intimacy, and managing social relationships might also require assistance.

Again, as with academic challenges, focusing on specific verbal and then written process-making is likely to be a worthwhile experiment. See Table 13.2 for additional information.

Choosing a college and vocation will also potentially be problematic and require thoughtful consideration. Jane Mcclure (in *Treating NVLD in Children, Broitman & Davis* 2013) offers practical suggestions for advising college-bound students both in how to choose the best learning environment and how to deal with admissions tests and the application process. C.M. Brown (in *Treating NVLD in Children*, Broitman & Davis 2013) covers the support offered and needed when actually attending college specifically emphasizing how to self-advocate and how to think

Table 13.2 Independent living skills

Daily routines	Regular sleep cycles, medication adherence, keeping a calendar, navigating public transit
Personal hygiene	Oral/hair/skin care, changing clothes, wearing deodorant
In case of emergency	Location of local hospital, important phone numbers, evacuation plan
Communication	How to send letters/postcards, writing a professional email, starting conversations with new people/strangers
Food preparation	Cooking and following a recipe, food storage, knife skills/safety, kitchen cleanliness
Finances	Paying bills/writing checks, credit vs. debit, avoiding ID theft, students loans, taxes
Communal living (i.e., dorms)	Sharing spaces with others, cleaning responsibilities, how to resolve differences
Basic home maintenance	Changing light bulbs, plunging a toilet, hanging a picture, flipping the breaker
Personal information	Practicing a signature, location of important documents (SS card, LD paperwork, birth certificate, passport), memorizing SS number
Illness	Finding and choosing a doctor understanding of OTC medications, basic first aid, understanding the differences between mild and serious illness
Laundry	Washing clothes/changing bed linens regularly, clothing care (ironing and dry cleaning), understanding washer and dryer settings, basic sewing repair
Dating and managing social relationships	Gender identity, sexual preference and sexuality, Safe sex practices, Dating etiquette and using dating apps, Internet security online presence and safety

Table 13.3 Colleges which include social support

Adelphi University, NY – Bridges Program (mentions NVLD) Dean College, MA – Arch Program (mentions NVLD) Manhattanville College, NY, Pathways and Connections (ASD and related diagnoses)
McDaniel College, MD – Mentorship Advantage Program
University of Denver, CO – Learning Effectiveness Program
Specific LD colleges
Landmark College – VT
Beacon College – FL

about the transition from college to career. Careful consideration is required to find the best fit between your patient's strengths and skills and interests, minimizing potential areas of challenges. Consult Table 13.3 for colleges which include social support programs and/or mention NVLD.

Should your patient prefer to join the workforce following high school, Lynn Koch (in *Treating NVLD in Children*, Broitman & Davis 2013) addresses the path to successful employment including job seeking skills and training.

13.4 Breaking Down Each Problem

Therapists need to get very detailed and specific with patients in order to diagnose the multitude of issues each problem contains, and there will be many! An example of one creating a decision-making checklist for a common problem related to how your patient might decide if they should attend an upcoming social event can be found in Appendix 8. These criteria are specific for the common sensory issues around light, heat, and sound. There may be additional concerns for your particular patient, and the two of you can and should customize decision-making checklists as needed. In the next chapter, we describe HomeWork Therapy™, a psychological treatment designed specifically for children with learning disorders and specifically NVLD.

References

Brown, C., & Leary, B. (2013). Coaching: Addressing the psychosocial and executive functioning challenges of NVLC in K-12 and their transition to adulthood. In J. Broitman & J. M. Davis (Eds.), *Treating NVLD in children: Professional collaborations for positive outcomes*. New York: Springer.

Koch, L. (2013). Employment and vocational rehabilitation with individuals with NVLD. In J. Broitman & J. M. Davis (Eds.), *Treating NVLD in children: Professional collaborations for positive outcomes*. New York: Springer.

Mcclure, J. (2013). College counseling with the NVLD student. In J. Broitman & J. M. Davis (Eds.), *Treating NVLD in children: Professional collaborations for positive outcomes*. New York: Springer.

Sensory-Processing-Disorder.com

Chapter 14
The Brooklyn Learning Center Model

14.1 HomeWork Therapy

Like all of the treatment approaches described throughout this book, HomeWork Therapy is delivered as part of a team approach. It requires collaboration with families, school faculty, tutors, therapists, speech/language pathologists, occupational, and physical therapists. Such communication is essential to ensure the child's success, as the challenges faced by children with NVLD often cut across domains and settings.

Our work with individuals with learning disorders starts from a core belief that learning disorders are neurodevelopmental disorders, consistent with where they are located in the DSM5. We also theorize that clinical components of learning disorders will respond to psychological intervention separately from educational interventions. We propose that individuals with NVLD require psychological interventions as a result of having NVLD in and of itself, not because NVLD may be comorbid with another psychological condition.

In our view, treatment for NVLD must address simultaneously the academic, cognitive, and emotional deficits inherent in NVLD and in all learning disorders. This psychological approach to treating learning disorders, including NVLD, has been developed over the past 20 years at the Brooklyn Learning Center by one of the authors (Margolis). The specific treatment is called HomeWork TherapyTM and combines psychotherapy with tutoring and cognitive remediation into a single treatment modality. Twenty years ago this psychological approach to learning problems was very rare, and people often were surprised that psychologists were providing such services. Now, however, with tutoring having become a multibillion dollar industry, psychologists treating learning and academic problems are not nearly as rare.

J. Broitman et al., *NVLD and Developmental Visual-Spatial Disorder in Children*, https://doi.org/10.1007/978-3-030-56108-6_14

HomeWork Therapy synthesizes knowledge from the medical, psychological, and educational fields into a single treatment modality. HomeWork Therapy incorporates treatment approaches designed by our team and also draws on existing evidence-based treatments to address specific aspects of each child's unique profile. For children with NVLD, these evidence-based interventions sometimes require modification to accommodate the visual–spatial deficits inherent in NVLD. We review some of how we address these issues in what follows.

HomeWork Therapy treatment is placed within the lexicon of play therapy, talk therapy, and behavioral therapy; homework is the medium in which we work, and we explore all of the usual aspects of therapy within this medium. When working with students with NVLD through HomeWork Therapy, therapists focus on improving academic and cognitive skills as well as psychological factors that affect learning and that are frequently associated with NVLD.

It is very important that students with NVLD leave sessions with completed homework assignments or, for lengthier assignments, a detailed understanding of and in-session practice completing parts of the task. For example, when a math assignment includes practice factoring quadratic equations using four different methods, we would first show the student that there are four different approaches needed and review each in words. Then we look together at the assignment and find one for each solution approach. We would then write out the solution approach for each type of problem, with annotated notes, capturing the students' own words for how they access the solution strategy. In this way we have created with the student a personalized approach to finishing homework. With time left in session, we would then have the student work to complete items in the assignment by applying the approaches written out above.

Importantly we help students develop a narrative such as First, what kind of problem is this? Second, which strategy can I use? I am not sure, so I will check each strategy starting with the first one. Or, I notice there is a coefficient (number) other than 1 defining the quadratic (squared) term, e.g., $3x^2$, so I will look for a strategy for solving equations with this form. Or, I am unable to find two numbers that multiply to the "c" term and add to the "b" term, so what can I do next? Ideally the sample guide has statements like this written out (or added as the session progresses), and the student can then decide to use complete the square or quadratic formula methods.

The gist of the approach is not *how* we teach solving quadratic equations but how we help students, in session, to generate strategies that they can use later, on their own or with a parent, teacher, or tutor. This requires a one-on-one interaction, listening to how students see problems, understanding what they think, and helping them to develop a tool that they can apply when the therapist is not present. It also requires utilizing our psychological understanding of the student to address any underlying issues also impacting them such as shame, self-esteem, or hopelessness. It is of critical importance that the therapist can seamlessly shift between modalities within a session, even midway through an exercise, and in response to the socio-emotional needs of students. The psychological context is therefore critical to success of the intervention.

HomeWork Therapy must be delivered by individuals who have training in how to be attuned to students' verbal and nonverbal communication. The psychological nuance and relationship are at the crux of the intervention. In our view, for students with NVLD (but also with any LD), this psychological nuance can only be achieved by entering the space (academic material, social interaction) where the student is challenged, thus requiring treatment to include working with and developing academic as well as psychological skills. By helping students in this manner, assignments get completed and/or positive social interactions increase, and ultimately school performance and life satisfaction often improve. This fosters success, which improves motivation, and the likelihood that the student will generalize these strategies to other situations at a later date increases.

Completing homework provides a useful outcome at the end of each session; leaving a session knowing that something difficult has been accomplished leaves students feeling good about the work, which is often challenging, and this in turn helps to reduce any resistance to treatment. Moreover, treatment does not place an additional burden on the student's time, which for those with NVLD is often very overburdened. Multiple outside treatments (social skills experiences, occupational therapy, etc.) often account for much of a student's after-school time. It is therefore critical that cognitive treatment helps students accomplish the demands of school while simultaneously addressing core cognitive deficits. This sounds like a daunting task, but neuropsychologists are expert at understanding how different cognitive abilities contribute to the execution of academic skills and activities and can thus use any assignment as a remediation tool. The overarching principal is to also make sure the student understands the approach or the how or why for doing something a particular way. Helping them identify their psychological triggers also empowers them to stop and reflect upon what is going on inside them. In this manner therapists will help students develop their own repertoire of strategies for approaching skills.

We are frequently asked: Does this help the student with NVLD improve their visual–spatial ability? This is an age-old question that requires much more research attention. If a student with dyslexia learns to read, is the phonological deficit that caused the dyslexia remediated, or has the student learned ways to execute phonological tasks? The extant empirical evidence is equivocal on this issue. Even less well understood is whether brain plasticity contributes to rewiring of core circuits (e.g., the student with dyslexia rewires the phonological circuit, or the student with NVLD rewires the spatial circuit) or by using alternative strategies compensatory mechanisms develop in the brain. Imaging studies of effects of treatment for dyslexia are plagued by methodological weaknesses (Bishop, 2013); however, they do suggest that both processes occur. No studies have examined functional or structural changes in the brain of children with NVLD before and after an intervention. Randomized controlled trials that include neuroimaging measures to assess change are required to further develop and test existing approaches for remediating visual–spatial deficits (Carretti, Lanfranchi, & Mammarella, 2013; Mammarella, Caviola, Cornoldi, & Lucangeli, 2013).

Addressing the academic, cognitive, and psychological aspects of NVLD in one treatment modality acknowledges the range of difficulties that are commonly associated with NVLD. As we have said throughout this book, a core deficit in visual–spatial processing is not isolated to functional impairment in visual–spatial skills. We espouse a "cognitive efficiency" model which theorizes that a core deficit in one area can have downstream effects on many other domains of function. As detailed in Chap. 2, Figs. 2.4–2.8, such downstream effects are often viewed as core deficits in the downstream domain, rather than as sequela of the true deficit. In Fig. 2.4, we show how a core deficit in visual–spatial ability may be interpreted as a deficit in social functioning, for example. Because HomeWork Therapy can address simultaneously the academic, cognitive, and psychological challenges common to NVLD, students and families feel committed to treatment, which can lead to treatment being high on the family and student's priority list. We routinely work with students for many years; this is not because students do not improve. Rather, each year students master the current expectations, but when they return the next year to school, there are new expectations to be met. Most often when students go to college, they are able to manage without us, typically because even if the expectations for time management and studying increase with the transition to college, the strategies that students have in combination with fewer demands on their time (college versus high school schedule) allow for success.

When engaging in HomeWork Therapy, in addition to applying our principles of the treatment, clinicians use a mix of evidence-based approaches from special education and psychology to deliver interventions that target the student's academic and psychological challenges. For some students with comprehension issues, for example, we might use Lindamood Bell Visualization–Verbalization to help students develop an image in their mind's eye of what they have read (a common problem for students with NVLD is that they do not do this automatically). Students with NVLD also frequently experience anxiety or obsessive compulsive disorder (OCD). In these cases, we use evidence-based best practice to treat the symptom. Sometimes these evidence-based treatments require modification for students with NVLD. For example, evidence-based therapies for anxiety and OCD have been well documented in the past decade. However, visualization, imagery, and sequencing underlie many components of these evidence-based treatments.

When an individual has a spatial deficit, this can affect how they can engage in treatment. For example, mindfulness is a powerful tool used in many evidence-based therapies; patients are instructed to conduct mindful observation of their thoughts. Many mindfulness strategies ask patients to use all five senses, including sight, to bring them into the present moment. This kind of visual mindfulness challenges the visual–spatial deficits that characterize NVLD. Similarly, when we teach coping skills, we often rely on visualization and imagery. We say to patients: imagine yourself in a place that makes you feel happy or calm. These are but a few ways that evidence-based practices require modification for use with individuals who have NVLD.

Regardless of whether the specific symptom requiring treatment is more academic or emotional, there are elements of it that will best be addressed with a psychological approach. HomeWork Therapy is a psychological treatment that requires training in the principles of psychotherapy to be delivered effectively. Below we describe the psychological aspects of treatment.

14.2 Psychological Support

In HomeWork Therapy for children with NVLD, the therapeutic alliance is specific to NVLD. Children with NVLD often receive subtle but painful feedback from their environment that they see the world differently from how others see it. They may feel as if their way of thinking is not accepted by others and receive feedback that what they do is "wrong" or "bad" (Palombo, 2001). In HomeWork Therapy, students with NVLD have the opportunity to experience working with a clinician who conveys an understanding of how the student sees the world, and so the student can come to trust the clinician. This feeling of being understood can also help students develop a cohesive sense of self. In HomeWork Therapy, the clinician attempts to understand the student's way of thinking before introducing a new concept or teaching an alternative approach, thereby eliminating the potential rejection of the student for their way of thinking. This experience is validating and helps the student feel accepted and valued.

Many students with NVLD experience shame and feel stigmatized for needing help. HomeWork Therapy aims to shift the locus of failure off of the student with NVLD in at least two ways. First, we work from the premise that in session the student's job is not to learn presented information but rather that the clinician's job is to make material accessible. When we first meet students, we often tell them: "At school you and your classmates sit and listen to the teacher. It is set up so that it is the teachers job to teach and it is your job to learn. Here, in our sessions your only job is to tell me when I am not teaching in a way that you can learn. The job is mine to teach in a way that makes sense; it is not your job to make sure you get it. Your only job is to tell me when you don't get it so that I can change my approach." This removes blame from the student and helps the student conceptualize difficulties within the context of their environment.

For some students and families, going to work with a tutor can feel more comfortable than seeing a therapist; a psychologist working within the HomeWork Therapy modality can explore and address emotional issues (i.e., social difficulties, low self-esteem) within the context of an academic treatment model. Second, HomeWork Therapy treatment aims to restructure cognitive schemas so that the student has positive, successful learning experiences. This ameliorates feelings of deficiency that are typically associated with learning (Palombo, 2001). In this way HomeWork Therapy can foster a positive transference to learning that may be generalized to other learning experiences outside of sessions, and the student develops a positive sense of self as a learner.

Many children with learning disorders are told that they cannot succeed due to neurobiological factors that are fixed and unchanging, and so they feel that they are just "not smart" (Palombo, 2001). Our approach to treatment shifts the focus from what is not malleable to what is. It teaches skills and strategies to help students understand that they are not broken and that they have the tools to be successful; they just need help mobilizing those tools. By taking these steps, HomeWork Therapy also aims to improve a sense of mastery by focusing on process and not on product which improves motivation (Dweck, 2006). But additionally, we are psychologists engaging in treatment, and the importance of the relationship permeates the delivery of the academic and cognitive interventions. The HomeWork therapist is always taking stock of the nature of the communication *during instruction* in order to understand the student's psychological makeup and helps build positive transference to learning or to develop new ways of communicating. The ability to flexibly shift from a tutoring modality to a therapy modality is an implicit part of the HomeWork Therapy approach. Without this and without implicit attention paid to how the child perceives the session, receiving help, showing what is hard for them, change is elusive.

When engaging in HomeWork Therapy, clinicians use a mix of approaches that draw from special education, neuropsychology, and psychology to deliver interventions that target a student's academic and psychological challenges. The case study below illustrates how this was achieved with a middle school girl.

Tawney's mother called our clinic at her wit's end. She reported that Tawney struggled throughout her final year of elementary school, and she was very concerned about her upcoming transition to middle school. She was planning to attend a prestigious middle school known for their challenging academic curriculum. She described Tawney as a bright, insightful preteen who struggled with understanding nuance in instructions and with being overly concrete in her thinking style. She reported that Tawney's struggles were highlighted at home because she internalized her difficulties, struggled to accept help, and frequently got down on herself for not understanding material. Her negative self-judgements would start what she termed the "Homework Wars" when Tawney would spend hours first avoiding her assignments and fighting with her parents and then staring at the page refusing to accept help and saying horrible things about her ability to finish her work. Tawney had been in therapy before to manage anxious feelings in early elementary school and had worked with tutors in the past. According to her mother, both of these experiences were objectively helpful, but Tawney found the act of participating in them painful.

Tawney's family provided me with detailed information about her feelings and behaviors provided her previous neuropsychological assessment, completed several years prior. According to this assessment, Tawney had superior working memory, verbal, and fluid reasoning abilities, but she struggled with visual–spatial understanding, motor coordination, processing speed, and attention. In short, Tawney was an exceptionally bright, capable student who worked more slowly than others and struggled with processing and manipulating visuospatial information and novelty. These challenges had taken an emotional toll on Tawney's ability to feel confident as a learner and had aggravated her anxiety. At the time of the evaluation, Tawney's difficulties were diagnosed as unspecified neurodevelopmental and anxiety disorder as well as a diagnosis capturing her motor challenges. To the HomeWork therapist, these data and her developmental course thus far suggested a nonverbal learning disability. Through this lens, the therapist was able to understand Tawney's challenges and explain them to her parents, to her school staff, and, most importantly, to her.

The therapist first met Tawney in September of her sixth-grade year. She was very hesitant to work with me because she believed her inability to get her work done independently spoke more to her failure as a student and less to her learning challenges. The therapist explained to Tawney that the work together would encompass homework help and that the therapist could help her work through things she didn't understand but more importantly that the therapist's goal was to help her understand why learning was so hard for her. She remained wary but agreed to give the therapist five sessions to see if the work together could be helpful.

The therapist used these first three sessions to help explain the concept of nonverbal learning disability to both Tawney and her family, as well as to give Tawney a chance to show the therapist what she felt she most needed help with. HomeWork Therapy allows clinicians to provide a mix of psychotherapy, remediation, and tutoring that flexibly shifts with each patient's needs. After gaining her trust, the therapist quickly discovered that tutoring would be the most minimal part of the work together. Instead, Tawney primarily struggled with understanding directions and would become fixated on small turns of phrase or unclear wording and would be unable to move past her concerns. Once she was started on an assignment and understood the directions, she was off like a rocket and completed assignments with ease.

The therapist began using the psychotherapy and cognitive remediation arms of the HomeWork Therapy model to help Tawney tolerate her uncertainty, practice asking for help, and improve her executive functioning skills. For example, the therapist started every session by reviewing the online homework portals for every class and writing assignments down in Tawney's school planner. The therapist also worked on modifying assignments to accommodate Tawney's learning challenges. Tawney struggled with engaging with her work on the computer because she would spend more time figuring out computer programs or trying to type out the perfect sentence than she would getting her ideas out on the paper. The therapist worked with Tawney's teachers to allow her to write assignments by hand and scan them into her email to turn them in. The therapist also worked on breaking down long-term assignments into smaller chunks, planning them out using outlines and graphic organizers, and getting started earlier to be able to implement her plan more efficiently. Each of these tasks was completed with graded practice – first, the therapist modeled the skills, and then they worked through the skills together, and then the therapist asked her to complete the skill on her own with supervision, before finally asking her to practice the skill at home on her own. Together, the therapist and Tawney communicated with her parents about the skills she was practicing so they could help remind her at any point if she became too overwhelmed to practice them on her own. Throughout this work, the therapist provided Tawney with psychoeducation about how anxiety can get in the way of schoolwork, cause procrastination, and make one feel bad about oneself. The therapist supplemented this psychoeducation with skills for recognizing thinking traps when Tawney came across complicated or confusing instructions and for helping her calm herself down and complete her work.

With those skills in place, Tawney flourished. She came prepared every week to sessions and transferred her new skills to homework time at home. There were still fights at home and her self-esteem was still growing, but her parents reported a meaningful difference in the time it took Tawney to complete her homework in the first 2 months of her work with her therapist. Shortly before winter break, Tawney began taking exams. She struggled to advocate for the extra time her Individualized Education Plan provided her because she was unwilling to make herself visible in front of her peers as "different" for using her accommodations. The therapist once again leaned on the HomeWork Therapy model to address Tawney's social anxiety and her negative core beliefs (e.g., asking for help means I'm stupid, if I don't get it the first time, I'm dumb and will never understand). Tawney and the therapist began writing emails to her teachers together, and the therapist was able to speak directly with her class advisor about the types of support she would most benefit from in the classroom. Opening these conversations allowed Tawney and the therapist to build Tawney's self-confidence, and she began to recognize that others also asked for help and clarification in the classroom. Her growing self-confidence in turn impacted her willingness to with engage her teachers and her grades improved.

By the end of the work, Tawney embraced the HomeWork Therapy model and all of her new skills. She began to complete her agenda before sessions, decide how the therapist could be most helpful to her, and advocate for the support she needed. These growing skills allowed the therapist to reinforce Tawney's growing self-confidence as she reflected on the progress she had made. This was highlighted most for her when she finished all of her final projects on time or early and with plenty of sleep the night before (compared to as much as 2 weeks late, just the semester before). Tawney's growing independence also allowed the therapist to rely less on parents' support for completing work at home, and the therapist and Tawney stopped sending weekly emails with skills updates. As a result, the therapist suggested family sessions to review the work. Through these sessions, Tawney's parents could learn how to help reinforce these skills in the future. Tawney agreed to take the reins, and after reviewing the executive functioning, anxiety, and procrastination skills she had gained, she taught those skills to her parents, with a focus on what worked best for her and how they could best support her in using those skills in the future.

Tawney received tutoring and therapy across various points in her development, but these models alone never quite addressed her needs. By combining these modalities within the HomeWork Therapy model, Tawney was able to access academic as well as therapeutic support in the moment of her greatest distress, doing homework. For the therapist, seeing her in an educational context was invaluable to understanding her learning disability and the interaction it had with her emotional distress. Doing academic work together allowed the therapist to build trust with Tawney and help her realize that she could seek help in a supportive, nonjudgmental environment without any negative connotations for her self-worth.

In the next Chap. 15, we offer guidelines and possible interventions to consider in the categories of visual–spatial, sensory perception, executive functioning, academics, social/emotional deficits, and motor coordination.

References

Bishop, D. V. (2013). Research review: Emanuel miller memorial lecture 2012 – Neuroscientific studies of intervention for language impairment in children: Interpretive and methodological problems. *Journal of Child Psychology and Psychiatry and Allied Disciplines, 54*(3), 247–259. https://doi.org/10.1111/jcpp.12034

Carretti, B., Lanfranchi, S., & Mammarella, I. C. (2013). Spatial-simultaneous and spatial-sequential working memory in individuals with down syndrome: The effect of configuration. *Research in Developmental Disabilities, 34*(1), 669–675. https://doi.org/10.1016/j.ridd.2012.09.011

Dweck, C. S. (2006). *Mindset: The new psychology of success*. New York: Random House.

Mammarella, I. C., Caviola, S., Cornoldi, C., & Lucangeli, D. (2013). Mental additions and verbal-domain interference in children with developmental dyscalculia. *Research in Developmental Disabilities, 34*(9), 2845–2855. https://doi.org/10.1016/j.ridd.2013.05.044

Palombo, J. (2001). *Learning disorders and disorders of the self in children and adolescents*. New York: WW Norton & Co.

Chapter 15
Specific Interventions

The major categories of deficits and dysfunction for children with NVLD can be usefully separated into *a primary deficit in visual–spatial processes and impairment in some functional domains including executive functioning, social/emotional deficits, and academic achievement and motor coordination.* There are also a host of ancillary difficulties that have been reported in NVLD, although how common these features remains unknown. Such clinical observations reflect difficulties with sensory perception, pragmatic language, part–whole relationships, managing novelty, and tactile processing to name a few. Future studies are required to more fully understand the complexities of the full clinical picture of NVLD.

Herein we discuss the generalizable principles, approaches, and attitudes we recommend using with students with NVLD. Additionally, when feasible, we describe interventions that have been mentioned as potentially helpful for each of these categories. We remind the reader that few if any of these interventions have an empirical basis. We have learned of these interventions through clinical anecdote, feedback from parents and schools, workshops, and educational meetings. These interventions are not endorsed by us but are offered to create a shared knowledge base of interventions and engender future research programs. Lastly, we will discuss the use of psychotherapy for children with NVLD.

15.1 General Principles/Approaches/Attitudes Toward Students with Nonverbal Learning Disabilities

We find it critical to avoid figures of speech and be literal. Children with NVLD often have trouble interpreting metaphors and may grow emotional in response to them. At minimum, they tend not to admit that they have not understood the figurative language. When working with students with NVLD, if they exhibit a behavior that you do not want/like, do not assume that this is a "character flaw" or "bad

J. Broitman et al., *NVLD and Developmental Visual-Spatial Disorder in Children*, https://doi.org/10.1007/978-3-030-56108-6_15

behavior." It will be more helpful to assume that it is likely a misunderstanding or miscommunication and then approach the child with that mindset. Assume their "Why …" questions are literal questions. Answer them literally before continuing to respond as you would to a child without NVLD.

As Russell Barkley (2005) has stressed for children with ADHD, every day is a new day. Holding grudges and creating resentment over the long term is likely to interfere with the relationship. Instead help lay out causes and effects, especially but not limited to the social ones. Mistakes made yesterday don't necessarily lead to progress tomorrow if one cannot understand the effects of one's actions, on self or on others. Children with NVLD have more difficulty than average with constructing sequences. For example, there are at least 50 steps involved in getting to their next appointment on time: hear bell in class, put books away, remember to take backpack, leave class, turn left, go downstairs, go to the bus stop, find the right bus, remember to pick up backpack, find seat, put backpack down, get off at the right stop (with backpack!), enter the building, and find the correct room. Observe the child's behavior closely, especially in novel or complex situations. We believe that the child's actual behavior should be our guide to understanding his or her struggles. It is generally understood that the new or novel situations will most likely generate the greatest problems for the child with NVLD. Directly observing the child will allow the professional to develop an intervention plan that focuses more specifically on the needed skills.

Teach the child in a systematic "step-by-step" fashion – we caution that it is easy to misjudge the child's capacity to take in information. Their superior verbal skill often leads professionals to overestimate the child with NVLD's overall skills and abilities. Instruction needs to be broken down and expressed verbally in simple sequential rules that the child can follow even though they have these verbal abilities. Teach the child appropriate strategies for dealing with particularly troublesome situations that occur on a frequent everyday basis. Rourke notes that generalization is difficult for children with NVLD, and specific detailed step-by-step solutions will be helpful. Teach appropriate nonverbal behavior – Rourke suggests the professional teach the child with NVLD how specifically to do it. He reminds us that the child often does not know when to smile, when not to smile, when to move, where to look, etc. He recommends the use of a mirror or video equipment that can allow a detailed analysis of behavior.

15.2 Major Categories of Challenges

15.2.1 Visual–Spatial (Core Deficits)

It is important for teachers and treatment professionals to recognize that there may sometimes be limitations in the child's/adolescent's visual, perceptual, and/or sensory processing modalities. They may be less "in sync" whenever material is presented in a purely visual modality.

Instructions with visual tasks should be verbally broken down in a logical step-by-step fashion. When something is presented in a visual or multimodal format, it should be accompanied by verbal cues and/or explanations. Keep in mind that the child will likely appreciate and benefit from, not tire of, lengthy, concrete verbal instructions and/or examples.

The child/adolescent may have difficulty "seeing the big picture" or the context from which details are extracted. While most people take a whole–part–whole approach to learning novel material, children and adolescents with these issues tend to take a part–whole approach, whereby they can become easily stuck in the details. These children/adolescents tend to benefit from assistance in "stringing" the details together to form the whole, which should be facilitated by the integration of step-by-step verbal instructions.

Teach the child to utilize verbal mediation for problem-solving. Try to make cause-and-effect relationships verbally explicit whenever possible. Try to demonstrate how details are part of a larger whole and/or how details can be grouped together as part of a whole, e.g., words may be grouped into categories within a larger list. The child can be overwhelmed by large amounts of materials; thus information should be presented in small "chunks" whenever possible. Large amounts of material, information, and homework assignments that have not been structured for them may be counterproductive given that they could become overwhelmed and distractible when so challenged. Teach the child/adolescent to use their verbal strengths to mediate their experiences. Verbal mediation is a powerful tool for these youngsters. Rely on their verbal strengths to teach decision-making, goal setting, and making action plans to achieve goals and evaluate results. Try to make the demands for performance as reasonable as possible, i.e., make sure demands are not overwhelming.

Teach and practice organizational skills. Utilize structure, routine, and rote or "scripted" rules when necessary to help the child/adolescent better manage situations. Teach the child/adolescent to self-monitor their own understanding of situations/instructions and to ask clarifying questions when necessary. Teach the child to make better use of his or her visual–perceptual–organizational. We caution professionals to help the child to exercise and develop his or her less developed skills to work toward achieving the highest level possible through age-appropriate remedial exercises. Teach the child to use age-appropriate aids to reach a specific goal. These may include digital watches, calculators, laptops, and various forms of assistive technologies which could be utilized to help improve the child's performance.

15.2.2 Visual–Spatial Processes

As we have stressed, children with NVLD often have a lack of image formation, poor visual recall, and faulty spatial perceptions. "They may get lost easily, or have difficulty finding things that are in plain sight. They may not be able to tell their left from their right" (Judy Lewis, NLDline). Interventions related to visual–spatial processes interventions can be found in Table 15.1.

Table 15.1 Visual–spatial processes

Interventions for visual–spatial processes
1. Optometric exercises – David Gresham's method (Griffin and Gresham (Griffin & Gresham, 2002)) to improve the eye tracking system
2. Direct instruction through educational therapy/tutoring
3. Photography classes – by learning how to capture visual images on paper, a child can develop better perception (Martin, 2007)
4. *The Source for Visual-Spatial Disabilities* (2002) by Neff, Neff-Lippman, and Stockdale offers suggestions to help learning to drive (Martin, 2007)
5. Juggling (Draganski, 2004) – In the study, published in the January 22 issue of *Nature*, researchers divided a group of young adults who had no experience in juggling into two groups. One group was given 3 months to learn how to juggle three balls simultaneously, and the others remained non-jugglers. MRI scans were performed at the start of the study, after the jugglers became skilled performers and could juggle for at least 60 s, and 3 months later. During that 3-month period, the jugglers did not practice or attempt to extend their skills. Although the participants had similar brain scans at the start of the study, the second scan revealed that the jugglers experienced significant expansion in the area of the brain associated with the processing and storage of complex visual motion. The amount of expansion also correlated with the juggler's performance. The more skilled they became, the greater growth they experienced. The increased areas seen on brain scans (among the jugglers) declined by the third brain scan. The non-jugglers showed no change in brain structure during the study Researchers say the temporary brain structure changes occurred in motion-selective areas of the brain, and the mechanism behind these changes is unclear and merits further study. Although this study was done with neurotypical participants, one author's anecdotal experience teaching juggling to children with NVLD suggests that it could be helpful (with a much longer training period involved). These changes are unclear and merit further study. Although this study was done with neurotypical participants, one author's anecdotal experience teaching juggling to children with NVLD suggests that it could be helpful (with a much longer training period involved)

15.3 Executive Functioning

Children with NVLD often have problems with organization which includes decision-making, planning, initiative, assigning priority, sequencing, motor control, emotional regulation, problem-solving, planning, impulse control, establishing goals, monitoring results of action, self-correcting, working memory, and problems with spatial relations. See Table 15.2 for executive functioning interventions.

15.4 Social/Emotional Challenges

Children with NVLD often have difficulties comprehending nonverbal communication "such as facial expression, body language, and tone of voice. They may not process efficiently and/or understand shrugs, winks, grins, or wrinkled foreheads. They may have trouble adjusting to transitions and novel situations, along with

Table 15.2 Executive functioning interventions

Executive functioning interventions
Behavior Rating Inventory of Executive Function™ (BRIEF®) Intervention manual by Gerard A. Gioia, PhD; Peter K. Isquith, PhD; Steven C. Guy, PhD; and Lauren Kenworthy, PhD. The BRIEF consists of three rating forms – a parent questionnaire, a child self-report, and a teacher questionnaire – designed to assess executive functioning in the home and school environments and a manual. The BRIEF might have been used to identify your patients' challenges. The manual offers behavior interventions geared to the results of the rating scale
Skills for School Success (Archer and Gleason, Curriculum Associates Inc.; 4th Printing edition January 1989)
Landmark Organizational Skills (Joan Sedita Landmark Study Skills Guide, Learning Disabilities: Information and Resources Landmark Foundation (September 1989)
The Kurzweil Study Skills Guide, and Teaching the Language Arts Tutorial Spectronics (2006) www.spectronicsinoz.com
Individual tutoring with organization therapist (e.g., in Northern California: SOS skills for success-www.sos4students.com Beth Samuelson)
Software programs such as Inspiration®, Kidspiration® (Inspiration Software 2008), and Don Johnston's Draft Builder (www.donjohnston.com) help students develop report ideas using webs, which are then converted into outline form

deficits in social judgment such as difficulty gauging appropriate personal space and social interaction" (Thompson, 1997).

Palombo (2006) recommends that the child be explicitly taught about nonverbal communications including facial expressions, gaze, body posture, vocal intonation, tactile communication, and proximity. We provide examples of how to accomplish this below. He also recommends that the clinician prepare the child for new situations by offering rehearsals or role-plays, encouraging integration of all aspects of stories. He views social cognitive impairments as a significant area of deficit for children with NVLD and recommends that they be taught social skills and strategies for understanding nonverbal communication in conjunction with mindsharing skills. By this he means that the child needs to be helped to speculate regarding why people take specific actions.

The clinician must try to discuss empathy with the child, to teach social functioning, and to encourage the development of a sense of humor. Palombo (2006) suggests that these things can be accomplished by having the clinician identify behaviors verbally, model behaviors to be learned, rehearse/practice potential actions/reactions with the child, and teach verbal mediation strategies. It will also be important to discuss and deal with feelings and to help the child to identify (decode) and express appropriate emotions. Palombo (2006) wants to help the child learn to mediate emotional states, in part by debriefing him or her following activities in order to help manage the anxiety in the moment.

Traditional social skills training programs, captured by phrases like friendship groups or playgroups, have not been found to be successful for children with NVLD without adjusting the intervention to address the types of perceptual and inferential thinking problems found with this diagnosis (Semrud-Clikeman & Schaefer, 2000). Semrud-Clikeman and Fine (2015) point out that one of the main issues with most social skill programs is that they begin at a level that does not directly train interpretation of facial expressions and body language. They feel that direct teaching of social perception skills through practice, modeling, and role-playing is likely most helpful. Teaching social perception through task analysis and rule teaching allows the child with NVLD to verbally process the information and use their strengths to learn new skills. They go on to say that the intervention needs to progress slowly with plenty of structure and time for the child to practice foundational skills before moving on to the more complex activities that require the building of trust in order to attempt them. For generalization of skills to occur, parent and teacher involvement are important in order to allow for practice of newly learned skills (Semrud-Clikeman, Fine, & Bledsoe, 2010).

15.5 Principles for Intervention

Those who are competent in the social arena are skilled at social executive functioning. In every environment, we have a social goal. In order to be successful in accomplishing our goal, we need to be able to do the following:

Plan – The ability to see what steps are required to manage the current and future social tasks and goals.

Initiate – The ability to independently begin the task and to generate ideas.

Monitor – Social dynamics are a rapidly changing landscape and what is required are the skills to perceive small changes in the social environment.

Shift – The ability to change your plan and even your goal depending upon the social information you receive.

Emotional control – The ability to modulate emotional responses and bring rational thought to bear on feelings. Poor judgment.

Self-monitor – The ability to monitor your own performance and to measure it against some standard of what is expected.

Some children with NVLD (often when comorbid with ADHD) are impulsive and tend to see only extremes as choices, missing the "gray zone." Therefore, helping them to slow down enough to consider gray areas can be very helpful, especially in social situations where the options generally are quite a bit more complex than "fight or surrender," "win or lose." The child's/adolescent's tendency to get stuck in the details of social events can be anxiety provoking, and once started this cycle may tend to escalate. The best way to deal with escalating frustration is to utilize relaxation techniques that can be used immediately when the frustration cycle begins. These techniques should be practiced often and in non-anxiety-provoking situations as well. Once the child/adolescent masters this technique, it can be applied to numerous situations that cause them anxiety or distress. Further, once relaxed, one can better learn to switch strategies and take an alternative strategy to a novel situation.

The child's/adolescent's nonverbal weaknesses can cause social difficulties and possible misperceptions. They may have trouble reading nonverbal cues, especially when they are subtle, and may have difficulty knowing how to respond in novel social situations. It is important to understand that the child may not accurately perceive the "gestalt" in social situations as well and might require assistance in the same step-by-step manner. They will likely do better in more highly structured social situations, but social skills training can help to better adapt to less structured situations.

Help the child develop insight into situations that are easy for him or her and those that are particularly troublesome. Here we stress the importance for the child [or adult] to understand his or her own cognitive functioning over time with the goal of developing a realistic understanding of his or her capacities. Once achieved, this understanding can help guide them to get assistance when needed and help them avoid situations that may be more likely to end in failure. It is also the cornerstone of self-advocacy. Anticipate the situations where they might have difficulty with transitions or novelty and provide advanced practice and support for how to deal with them. Teach the child/adolescent to self-monitor their own understanding of situations/instructions and to ask clarifying questions when necessary. See Table 15.3 for examples on how to create a self-monitoring intervention.

Table 15.3 Interventions for social/emotional challenges

Interventions for social/emotional challenges
Social Competence Intervention Program (Guli, Wilkinson, & Semrud-Clikeman, 2008) has been designed to work with children with NVLD and Asperger's disability. SCIP is an intervention that is multisensory in nature and targets underlying difficulties in social perception as well as providing exercises to improve the generating of strategies for problem-solving. The SCIP exercises were adapted from children's creative drama and theater classes and provide practice in developing an accurate perception and response to facial and vocal cues. The exercises move from perception of emotions to interpretation and then to response. Initially the child sees pictures of faces and with mastery of emotional recognition and labeling is presented with naturalistic vignettes of children interacting. As the child progresses through the program, they are introduced to understanding their own emotions and then those of others. The work is constantly reviewed and supported throughout the time of the intervention, thus providing for review and refreshing of skills. The activities that are part of SCIP are reported by the children to be fun. Guli (2005) evaluated the efficacy of the SCIP program. In this study, the children improved in their ability to correctly recognize facial expressions as well as vocal cues following the intervention. Qualitative results showed that 75% of parents reported one or more positive changes in social perception or competence after participating in the intervention, while 82% of the children reported one or more positive effects of the intervention. Thus, this study's results suggest that effects may generalize over settings (i.e., home and school). The results of this study lend support to the efficacy of the SCIP program that targets specific difficulties in a very specialized population. Moreover, these findings strongly support research that stresses training in perception and integration of nonverbal cues for children with nonverbal learning disabilities (Barnhill, Cook, Tebbenkamp, & Myles, 2002)

(continued)

Table 15.3 (continued)

Interventions for social/emotional challenges
Parent Effectiveness Training (PET) and general programs for parental involvement (Gordan, 2006) have been used with children with NVLD. In addition to these manualized programs, parents are recommended to provide opportunities for their child to participate in organized activities such as Boy or Girls Scouts, 4-H, and other structured experiences. In cases where the family has social difficulties, family therapy has often been recommended (Carlson & Christenson, 2005). While some parents may not be temperamentally or experientially able to appropriately teach social skills, it is helpful to provide information about resources, developmental progress, and interventions
Michelle Garcia Winner – Center for Social Thinking – www.socialthinking.com provides training, workshops, and curriculum for social skills training
The Social Emotional Learning Framework (SELF): A way to enhance understanding and focus interventions, the SELF was developed by Meryl Lipton, M.D., PhD, Director of Rush Neurobehavioral Center in Chicago Illinois and her team. The framework is presented as a possible way to help refocus clinical and research efforts regarding children with NVLD and other brain-based social emotional learning disabilities (BB-SELD). Rather than primarily being concerned with delineating differences among BB-SELD children, the SELF, instead, emphasizes their shared difficulties in processing social–emotional information. More specifically, the SELF describes (1) a possible set of brain-based social–emotional processes, (2) currently available ways to assess social emotional learning strengths and weaknesses, and (3) a variety of strategies for interventions
Speech therapists can help students with NVLD with both semantic and pragmatic language. An example of such a language program is Diamond Social Skills, created by Susan Diamond, M.A., CCC Speech Pathologist. It provides parents with activities, strategies, and games to help their children develop social skills. It discusses turn taking, topic initiation, language processing, etc. (www.diamondlanguage.com)
College Internship Program – Michael McManmon (www.Collegeinternshipprogram.com) offers a residential treatment program providing wrap around support for college students with NVLD
Comic Strip Conversations and Social Stories (Gray, 1994)
Helping the Child who Doesn't Fit In (Nowicki & Duke, 1992)
Teaching Your Child the Language of Social Success (Duke et al., 1992).
Navigating the Social World (McAfee, 2013)
Emotion cards and social games are available from Western Psychological Services, Creative Play Therapy division
Relationship Development Intervention (RDI) is a lifespan model, designed by Dr. Steven Gutstein, which is broken into stages that are appropriate for toddlers through adults. Information is available at the following website: http://www.rdiconnect.com/ also has a DVD available to help teach the recognition of emotions. It is available at the following website: www.human-emotions.com
Mind Reading: The Interactive Guide to Emotions (Baron-Cohen, 2004; www.jkp.com/mindreading). This is an interactive program that demonstrates over 400 different human emotions
Thinking Publications (Social Star) at www.thinkingpublications.com may be helpful
Teaching Your Child the Language of Social Success, by Marshal P. Duke, Stephen Nowicki Jr., and Elisabeth A. Martin (1996), is a book/manual for helping children and a follow-up book for adults as well (Nowicki & Duke, 1992) who have difficult reading or sending nonverbal emotional material (this is referred to as dyssemia) which works on improving verbal and nonverbal processing skills. There are ideas for working with individuals as well as adapting the principles to the classroom

(continued)

Table 15.3 (continued)

Interventions for social/emotional challenges
Watch sitcoms on television – Our clinical experience supports the use of repeated viewing together and discussion of comedy and soap opera television shows such as "Big Bang Theory" and "Third Rock from the Sun." The exaggerated emotions portrayed on these shows offers ample opportunity for discussion and increased understanding. Techniques such as practicing in front of a mirror, listening to recorded speech, watching a video recorded behavior, and so forth should all be incorporated. Watch with the sound off and work together to identify the facial expressions. Videotaping the child and reviewing the material together is an additional way to address these deficits
It is important to help the student develop the ability to make inferences, to predict, to explain motivation, and to anticipate multiple outcomes so as to increase the flexibility with which the student both thinks about and uses language
Directly teach the child/adolescent with NVLD to make eye contact and attend to and interpret facial expressions, gaze, gestures, prosody, vocal inflections, and other nonverbal aspects of communication. There are many different techniques to do this such as:
Using pictures – Take or gather photos of people your patient knows. Look for a range of facial expressions. Print and make flashcards. You can use them to:
Help your patient identify the feeling that goes with the expression on the card
Ask why your child thinks it's the right emotion
Each takes a card, and mimics the expression, and have the other person guess what it is
Name times you've seen someone make that facial expression
Ask your patient to find pictures in magazines or on websites of people whose expressions match those in the flashcards
Analyze facial features – Show how the eyebrows, mouth, eyes, nose, and forehead change with emotion. Practice making expressions like "angry eyes." Looking in the mirror can help kids see how accurate their expressions are
Analyze facial movement – Ask your patient to pay attention to what face muscles feel like when feeling happy, sad, angry, etc. Have kids look in the mirror to see each expression. That can help them see it in other people's faces
Help your patient notice changes – Point out the "neutral" faces of family members and friends. This can help them see changes in expression
Try out apps – There are many apps that teach emotions and facial expressions. These games are a fun way to practice recognizing facial expressions independently and discreetly
Teach kids to ask – Remind your child that it's OK to say something like "Sometimes I can't tell if you're mad. Are you?" Taken from: helping-your-child-learn-to-read-facial-expressions – https://www.understood.org/en/friends-feelings/common-challenges/picking-up-on-social-cues/helping-your-child-learn-to-read-facial-expressions
See for additional examples: Teaching-Facial-Expressions-of-Emotion.pdf
Create a self-monitoring intervention. Self-monitoring has two components, measurement and evaluation (Loftin, Gibb, & Skiba, 2005): That is, the student (1) measures and records his or her own behavior (measurement) and then (2) compares that recorded behavior to a predetermined standard (evaluation). Self-monitoring can take many forms. One student may use a paper form to rate her study skills at the end of each class period, for example, while another student might verbally rate his social behaviors when approached by his teacher at random times across the school day. The five steps involved in planning a self-monitoring intervention:
1. Identify the target behavior
2. Select/design a self-monitoring system
3. Choose reinforcers and how the student will earn them

(continued)

Table 15.3 (continued)

Interventions for social/emotional challenges
4. Teach the student to use the system
5. Fade the role of the adult in the intervention
These individualized plans are used to increase independent functioning in academic, behavioral, self-help, and social areas. Rather than focusing on reducing a student's undesired behavior, self-monitoring strategies develop skills that lead to an increase in appropriate behavior. When self-monitoring skills increase, corresponding reductions in undesired behaviors often occur, even without direct intervention (Dunlap, Clarke, Jackson, & Wright, 1995; Koegel, Harrower, & Koegel, 1999). This collateral behavior change allows teachers and parents to address multiple behaviors with one efficient intervention
Relaxation techniques – These are particularly valuable as they can be used immediately, anywhere, when the frustration cycle begins. Explore with your patient which of the many work best for them. Some examples are using a breath focus. In this simple, powerful technique, you take long, slow, deep breaths (also known as abdominal or belly breathing), body scan. This technique blends breath focus with progressive muscle relaxation as you work your way through each part of your body to check in and relax the muscles; there are also many forms of mindfulness meditation, yoga, tai chi, and qigong. These techniques should be practiced often and in non-anxiety-provoking situations as well

15.6 Intellectual Reasoning

Children with NVLD often have difficulty with reasoning, including visual–spatial reasoning and fluid reasoning/novel problem-solving. Intellectual reasoning interventions can be found in Table 15.4.

15.7 Academics

Academic interventions are often needed to support children with mathematics, writing, and planning/organization and reading comprehension.

15.8 Math

Interventions can consist of direct instruction and therapies, modification of classroom environment, modification of academic load, and scaffolding to support the student's progress in non-affected areas (Semrud-Clikeman, Fine, & Bledsoe, 2010). Written calculation was found to be most impaired (Forrest, 2004), suggesting that the mechanics of performing written math (i.e., lining up number columns) is an area of difficulty. Modifications to help with this problem include using graph or column paper to assist with number alignment. Adjustment of the curriculum to

Table 15.4 Intellectual reasoning interventions

Intellectual reasoning interventions
Perceptual Enrichment Program (PEP) – PEP (Kreidler, 1996) is a cognitive-based developmentally oriented treatment modality based on principles of both child development and cognitive rehabilitation. A trained therapist, most often an occupational therapist, who guides the child's exploration, presents novel, developmentally graded problem-solving tasks using the materials to tailor the task to the child's developmental and remedial needs. Materials include primary school activities such as mosaic designs, sorting, logic, and sequential reasoning tasks that encourage the child to integrate both analytical and gestalt problem-solving strategies. The Perceptual Enrichment Program, developed in 1982, has some clinical/anecdotal evidence suggesting that it can effect changes in skills thought to be mediated by frontal lobe development in a number of children treated both at the California Pacific Medical Center's Child Development Center (CMPC) and by occupational and educational therapists in private practice (Kreidler, 1996). To date, case studies utilizing PEP reveal changes in attention, visual perception, classification, processing speed, and visual–motor integration among a sample of school-aged children treated from 1993 to 1996 at CPMC (Kreidler, 1996). Changes of one to two standard deviations on standardized tests of cognitive processing were seen among students in a preliminary retrospective study (Kreidler, 1996, unpublished manuscript and personal communication). Geographically, the two main areas PEP associations can be found are in Copenhagen, Denmark, and in San Francisco, Ca., USA. It has also been reported that the PEP is currently being studied in Boston M with MRIs taken before and after PEP treatment by qualified facilitators. Information can be requested by contactingptheisen@mantraonline.com
Drawing with Language (www.lblp.com or 800 233-1819) is a structured program developed by Lindamood-Bell to improve visual spatial skills through their summer programs. Students are taught to visualize a math concept and then learn to draw it

include an enriched verbal explanation of the material as opposed to blackboard demonstration only has proven useful, by clinical report. While early number concepts and facts may not necessarily challenge children with NVLD, as concepts become more abstract and spatial (e.g., geometry, trigonometry), they may benefit from one-on-one tutoring by a mathematics educator skilled in translating math concepts verbally. Math interventions can be found in Table 15.5.

15.9 Writing

Writing is often an area of difficulty for children with NVLD. Initially, it is the physical act of writing which forms a barrier to developing writing as a method of effective communication (see the section on fine motor skills in this chapter). Dictation is often recommended for content-based exercises if the child is not able to produce a written product. By allowing the child to continue to grow academically without being held back by production issues, some negative emotionality and lowering of self-esteem may be avoided (Davis & Broitman, 2007). Older students may experience difficulty with organizing their ideas into a cohesive written report. If symptoms of ADHD are present, this type of task can become even more

Table 15.5 Math interventions

Math interventions
On Cloud Nine® (www.lblp.com or 800 233-1819) is a structured program developed by Tuley and Bell (1997), which stimulates the ability to image and verbalize the concepts underlying math processes. Concept and numeral imagery are integrated with language and applied to math computation and problem-solving. There is emphasis on both mathematical reasoning and mathematical computation
Math from A-Z – Sarah Harris (sarahha2z@sbcglobal.net). This is a color-coded, well-structured, and sequenced curriculum for basic math skill development. Originally intended as an instructional set of strategies with more verbalization meant to appeal more to girls, the added structure, strategy, and verbalizations could also be helpful to students with NVLD
Making Math Real – David Berg: A Multisensory, Structured Program for Cognitive Development in Mathematics (http://www.makingmathreal.org/). This program offers multisensory structured methodologies which delivers all instruction via the three processing modalities: visual, auditory, and kinesthetic–motoric. The creators of Making Math Real suppose that students who are struggling experience processing difficulties in either one or more of these processing modalities. They emphasize that best instructional practices require linking all incoming information across the three channels to maximize successful processing
Math-U-See (Demi, undated; http://MathUSee.com). This is another multisensory, manipulative-based curriculum for beginning math skills up through precalculus (including algebra and geometry). The program includes a series of DVDs and materials to enhance math skills in struggling students The approach includes:
Explicit instruction – directly teaches skills for math
Systematic and cumulative – has a definite logical sequence of concept introduction
Structured – uses step-by-step procedures for introducing, reviewing, and practicing concepts
Multisensory – engages visual, auditory, and kinesthetic channels simultaneously or in rapid succession
Progress monitoring – uses ongoing progress monitoring with frequent opportunities to reteach
There was one evaluation of the program noted on the website where students receiving special education services in the Albuquerque Public Schools demonstrated significant gains through the implementation of Math-U-See. However, there were no control group
5. Math apps:
1. Mathmagics offers a range of apps – see https://apps.apple.com/us/app/mathemagics-mental-math/id306586847
2. Algebra – Desmos and GeoGebra. Both allow you to drag points, lines, and circles around to see how they behave as the measure of angles and line segments changes: Desmos (https://www.desmos.com/calculator/dseyqv1dde)
GeoGebra (https://www.geogebra.org/?lang=en)
3. ModMath (http://www.modmath.com): the app displays virtual graph paper, which kids can use to set up math equations. Kids enter their equations, and the program aligns numbers and symbols in neat columns and/or rows so the equations are clearly legible. They save their worksheets and create PDFs to share or print
4. http://www.dyscalculia.org/math-tools

challenging (see the section on executive functioning in Chap. 7). Adolescents with NVLD may need more help from adults during this process than do their non-affected peers. Writing interventions can be found in Table 15.6.

Table 15.6 Writing interventions

Apps for writing:
The Writing Revolution – Judith C. Hochman and Natalie Wexler. Using The Writing Revolution method can be a way of ensuring NVLD students are grasping content and thinking analytically. Provides a clear method of instruction to use across grades and courses. May improve reading comprehension, improve organizational and study skills, enhance speaking abilities, and help develop analytical capabilities
(a) StoryBuilder: helps children (1) improve paragraph formation, (2) improve integration of ideas, and (3) improve higher-level abstractions by inference
(b) SimpleMind+: Mind mapping for any kind of writing project. Students use the app to brainstorm or organize ideas on a specific topic

15.10 Reading Comprehension

Many NVLD students are found to have receptive language challenges especially in the areas of pragmatic language. Others have written about how these difficulties can impact aspects of advanced reading skills which depend on such abilities, such as inferencing, summarizing, and saliency determination (Levine, 2002; Rourke & Tsatsanis, 1996; Worlng, Humphries, & Tannock, 1999). And again, these challenges can be remediated with direct and explicit reading comprehension instruction with some available programs listed below. Reading comprehension interventions can be found in Table 15.7.

15.11 Motor Coordination

Children with NVLD may need the assistance of an occupational therapist that can help the child develop fine and/or gross motor control. Such children often have poor fine and gross motor coordination, severe balance problems, and difficulties with graphomotor skills. They were probably late learning to tie their shoes or ride a bike – or they may never have learned at all. They may have trouble catching a ball. They may write slowly, and their handwriting may be illegible (Davis & Broitman, 2006). For handwriting, some (e.g., Martin, 2007) have found that moving from printing to handwriting early helps alleviate writing challenges for children with NVLD, while others (Berninger & Richards, 2002) say that if a child is having trouble printing, moving to cursive can create two dysfluent systems and that printing efficiency should be the focus. Both sets of researchers seem to agree that when the physical act of writing is severely challenging, moving the child to a keyboard-based or voice-activated system is advised. Motor coordination interventions can be found in Table 15.8.

Table 15.7 Reading comprehension interventions

Reading comprehension interventions
Lindamood-Bell Visualizing and Verbalizing® program (V/V®) attempts to stimulate the underlying process involved in reading to improve comprehension and to stimulate concept imagery. Individuals may become able to image gestalts that include color and movement. It has been found to improve their language comprehension, reasoning for critical thinking, and expressive language skills in some children. Although there is no research specifically designed for students with NVLD, their website does have research documenting the success of this program among children with other learning problems. However, we must be mindful that it was really developed for children with dyslexia rather than NVLD (visit www.lblp.com). It has been suggested BY Martin (2007) that its reliance on rules can be useful for our children with NVLD
Edzyme™ ("Educational Enzyme") model (http://www.individualu.com/) provides one-on-one mentor–tutors who are part of a collaborative student-centric educational team that communicates regularly with parents, schools, and therapists to help a child's progress
There are a number of books written to address students' difficulties with reading comprehension. Books such as *Bringing Words to Life* (Beck, McKeown, & Kucan, 2013), *Vocabulary Development* (Stahl, 1999), and *Improving Reading Comprehension: Research Based Principles and Practices* (Carlisle & Rice, 2002) are good examples. For a more comprehensive list of possible intervention-oriented books, see Martin (2007)
(a) StoryBuilder: helps children (1) improve paragraph formation, (2) improve integration of ideas, and (3) improve higher-level abstractions by inference
(b) SimpleMind+: mind mapping for any kind of writing project. Students use the app to brainstorm or organize ideas on a specific topic

Table 15.8 Motor coordination interventions

Motor coordination interventions
Occupational therapy/physical therapy – teaching movement with words
Loops and other groups: Kinesthetic Writing System (Benbow, 1999) Mary Benbow – emphasizes the motor skills needed to form letters
The grotto grip (www.grottogrip.com) is a plastic grip that attaches to a pencil to help a student learn the correct way to hold the pencil
Keyboarding skills (1986) – Diana King: helps the student learn the keyboard using verbal cues
Keyboarding instruction such as Type To Learn (https://www.typetolearn.app)
Handwriting Without Tears (www.hwtears.com) developed by Jan Olsen has been used with some success in the schools, by clinical report
Helping Children Overcome Learning Difficulties (Rosner, 1979) by Jerome Rosner offers specific suggestions on improving motor skills including The Visual Perception skills program which can be modified for children with NVLD
Games and activities that develop fine motor skills and visual perception such as juggling and drumming. May be borrowed through your local library or through the National Lekotek Center, www.lekotek.org
British style walkers help children with motor difficulties walk more stably (WWW.Galttoys.com)
The learning window (www.arkinst.org) allows one to demonstrate drawing facing the student
The Source for Visual Spatial Disorders (2002) by Neff, Neff-Lippman, and Stockdale include a chapter on how to learn to drive as well as deal with other spatial issues
Browns' (2005) *Helping the Learning Disabled Adolescent Learn to Drive* offers useful suggestions that can be adapted to students with NVLD (www.ldaamerica.org/aboutld/parents/help/drive.asp)

15.12 Psychotherapy

Finally, we would like to discuss group and individual psychotherapy and life coaching as potential interventions for our NVLD clients. Considerable controversy exists regarding the usefulness of these interventions. Research on the treatment of emotional and behavioral disturbances is needed to determine the appropriateness of different therapeutic approaches with this population. To this end, further study may attempt to identify the specific type of therapy that is best suited for individuals with NVLD. Although researchers suggest that insight-oriented therapy may appear to be indicated due to the verbal strengths of individuals with NVLD (Rourke & Tsatsanis, 1996), Schloerb (2005) reminds us that it is important to remember that a high level of verbal output does not equate with abilities in concept-forming and problem-solving, which can be significantly lacking in individuals diagnosed with NVLD. Specifically, she recommends that therapists must explore the ways in which therapy might capitalize on existing linguistic strengths in order to treat cognitive deficits. *Both Brett and Moira express appreciation for the role of therapy in their lives. Brett says "working with my therapist helped me immensely. His goal was to understand me; he spent a lot of time listening to me and trying to see all the factors that contributed to my struggles. His office felt like a sanctuary, where I felt the most free to honestly express my difficulties. I am enormously grateful and could never thank him enough for what he did for me."*

There is a general consensus in the field of learning disabilities that problems persist throughout the life cycle (Johnson, 1987; Palombo, 2001), suggesting that therapy may continue to be useful throughout or at least intermittently. Adults with NVLD have reported that counseling is helpful in dealing with frustration, but Schloerb (2005) suggests that practitioners should also include help for immediate problem-solving, rather than only emphasizing the resolution of previous conflicts (Johnson, 1987).

Due to the highly verbal nature of children with NVLD, the authors believe that therapy is likely to be helpful at least in some circumstances. It would be imperative that the clinician have familiarity with the particular characteristics of their clients with NVLD, such as their tendency toward concreteness, misinterpretation of pragmatics, difficulty with insight, and need for repeated practice prior to generalization. They should be well informed regarding the success of psychopharmacology with depression and anxiety reduction. The therapist can best function as a life coach providing a safe environment where the child/adult can verbally mediate their concerns and receive practical guidance. We have had considerable success working with the family as a whole, helping the child to express their needs and clarify expectations. Frequency of meeting is less important than available when the patient is experiencing distress. In addition, the therapist can use their dynamic understanding to help the child/adult with NVLD mediate developmental milestones and achieve maximum autonomy.

15.13 Nonverbal Communication Skills in Psychotherapy

As mentioned previously, children can have both NVLD and autism, potentially resulting in significant trouble with the nonverbal communication skills needed to form social connections (interpreting facial expression or vocal tone). In one author's clinical practice, consistent differences have been observed in the presentation of these social issues between patients with NVLD and patients who have both NVLD and autism. With our patients with NVLD, therapists, for example, may initially have difficulty understanding how their patient thinks in terms of their priorities, thought processes, and more. What is less likely to be an issue, however, is the feeling of having an emotional connection, as having NVLD social issues including mismatched facial expressions does not mean not having or expressing emotions or the desire to connect with others. People with NVLD are often considered "outgoing and friendly" and therefore presumed to want social communication but appear to have difficulty with the skills required to make social connections.

We hypothesize that for individuals with NVLD, these deficits make the assessment of when environments and situations may be ripe for forming social connections difficult. In addition, children with NVLD often have trouble matching their own facial expressions or tone of voice to a situation, so even if they can correctly identify a propitious situation, they may find it difficult to take advantage of this opportunity through appropriate and encouraging nonverbal behaviors. In contrast, a core feature of ASD is a deficit in social reciprocity. There are long-standing misperceptions that this means that children with autism do not have feelings or insights or want friendships/romance/interpersonal connections (Sedgewick et al., 2018). One reason for this impression may be relatively straightforward: children with autism appear to have difficulty conveying their internal emotional state outwardly, possibly through a decreased ability to automatically use and understand a variety of tones and facial expressions. To observers, therefore, it may appear that people with autism do not want social connections; because they have difficulty expressing this need as well as forming these connections, their lack of contact might be mistaken for or seen as a lack of desire for contact (Sala et al., 2020). For some of our patients with NVLD and autism, however, the presence of emotions internally might be less likely to be expressed visually or verbally to the outside, especially in new environments including with new people.

Our conjecture is that trying in therapy to connect first on an emotional level, as is common among neurotypicals, and may be effective for connecting with most NVLD patients, is less likely to be successful with our co-occurring diagnose patients. Given the vulnerability and hypersensitivity to discussing emotional issues, a comfortable place to begin building a connection with all of our patients may be in their areas of obsessive interests, which may also be a useful tactic to keep in mind if a patient, often a child with NVLD, also has deep and sustained niche interests. Some of their social difficulties, however, may be resolved through similar interventions and therapy. For example, similar types of interventions to improve the skill of interpreting others' facial expressions and tones as well as how to modulate and apply one's own facial expressions and tones of voice to engender bilaterally satisfying social communication may work for both or co-occurring diagnoses. Clearly, further research will be required to refine and answer these questions as they have treatment and intervention implications.

Our last chapter offers our closing thoughts. In this book, we have synthesized our suggestions for the best practices for treating children or adults with a nonverbal learning disability.

References

Archer, A, & Gleason, M. (1989, January). *Skills for school success associates Inc.* (4th printing ed., January). Curriculum Associates Inc.

Barkley, R. A. (2005). *ADHD and the nature of self-control*. New York: Guilford.

Barnhill, G. P., Cook, K. T., Tebbenkamp, K., & Myles, B. S. (2002). The effectiveness of social skills intervention targeting nonverbal communication for adolescents with asperger syndrome and related pervasive developmental delays. *Focus on Autism and Other Developmental Disabilities, 17*(2), 112–118

Baron-Cohen, S. www.human-emotions.com

Baron-Cohen, S. (1997). *Mindblindness: An essay on autism and theory of mind*. Cambridge, MA: MIT Press.

Baron-Cohen, S. (2004). *Mind reading: The interactive guide to emotions*. www.jkp.com/mindreading

Beck, I., McKeown, M., & Kucan, L. (2013). *Bringing words to life*. New York: Guilford Press.

Benbow, M. (1999). *Loops and other groups: Kinesthetic writing system*. Communication Skill Builders.

Berg, D. *Making math real- a multisensory*. (Structured Program for Cognitive Development in Mathematics). http://www.makingmathreal.org/

Berninger, V., & Richards, T. (2002). *Brain literacy for educators and psychologists*. Elsevier Science.

British style walkers help children with motor difficulties walk more stably. www.Galttoys.com.

Browns. (2005). *Helping the learning disabled adolescent learn to drive offers useful suggestions that can be adapted to students with NVLD*. www.ldaamerica.org/aboutld/parents/help/drive.asp

Carlisle, J., & Rice, M. (2002). *Improving reading comprehension: Research based principles and practices*. York Pr

Carlson, C., & Christenson, S. L. (2005). Evidence-based parent and family interventions in school psychology: Overview and procedures. *School Psychology Quarterly, 20*(4), 345–351. https://doi.org/10.1521/scpq.2005.20.4.345

Davis, J., & Broitman, J. (2006). A brief overview of nonverbal Learning disorders. *The Educational Therapist, 27*(3), 5–10.

Davis, J., & Broitman, J. (2007). Nonverbal learning disabilities: Models of proposed subtypes, part II. *The Educational Therapist, 27*(4), 5–10.

Demme Learning Math U See. http://MathUSee.com

Desmos. https://www.desmos.com/calculator/dseyqv1dde

Diamond, S. *Diamond social skills, created by Susan Diamond*. www.diamondlanguage.com

Draganski, B., Gaser, C., Busch, V., Schuierer, G., Bogdahn, U., & May, A. (2004). Neuroplasticity: Changes in grey matter induced by training. *Nature, 427*, 311–312.

Duke, M., & Nowicki. (1992, 1996). *Teaching your child the language of social success*. http://www.rdiconnect.com/

Dunlap, G., Clarke, S., Jackson, M., & Wright, S. (1995). Self-monitoring of classroom behaviors with students exhibiting emotional and behavioral challenges. *School Psychology Quarterly, 10*, 165–177.

Dyscalculia Remediation Programs. http://www.dyscalculia.org/math-tools

Forrest, B. (2004). The utility of math difficulties, internalized psychopathology, and visual spatial deficits to identify children with the nonverbal learning disability syndrome: Evidence for a visual-spatial disability. *Child Neuropsychology, 10*(2), 129–146. https://doi.org/10.1080/09297040490911131

Geogebra. https://www.geogebra.org/?lang=en

Gioia, G. A., Isquith, P. K., Guy, S. C., & Kentworthy, L. (2020). *Behavior rating inventory of executive function*. Lutz, FL: Psychological Assessment Resources, Inc.

Gordan, T. (2006). *Parent effectiveness training*. Solana Beach, CA: Gordon Training International.

Gray. (1994). *Comic strip conversations and social stories*. Arlington: Future Horizons. https://carolgraysocialstories.com/about-2/carol-gray/

Griffin, J., & Gresham, D. (2002). *Binocular anomalies: Diagnosis and vision therapy* (4th ed.). Oxford, UK: Butterworth-Heinemann.

Guli, L. A. (2005). The effects of creative drama-based intervention for children with deficits in social perception. *Dissertation Abstracts International Section A: Humanities and Social Sciences, 65*, (10-A).

Guli, L. A., Wilkinson, A., & Semrud-Clikeman, M. (2008). *Enhancing social competence on the autism spectrum: A drama-based intervention for youth*. Champaign, IL: Research Press.

Gutstein, S. (2002). *Relationship Development Intervention (RDI)*. London: Jessica Kingsley Publishers,

Harris, S. *Math from A-Z- Sarah.* sarahha2z@sbcglobal.net

helping-your-child-learn-to-read-facial-expressions

Hochman, J., & Wexler, N. (2017). *The writing revolution – A guide to advancing thinking through writing in all subjects and grades*. Jossey-Bass

Edzyme™ ("Educational Enzyme") model. http://www.individualu.com/

Inspiration®, Kidspiration®. (2008). *Inspiration Software*.

Johnson, D. J. (1987). Nonverbal disorders and related learning disabilities. In D. J. Johnson & J. Blalock (Eds.), *Adults with learning disabilities*. New York: Grune & Stratton, Inc.

Johnston, D. *Don's Johnston draft builder*. www.donjohnston.com

King, Diana, Keyboarding skills. (1987). *Helps the student learn the keyboard using verbal cues*. Educators Pub Service.

Koegel, L. K., Harrower, J. K., & Koegel, R. L. (1999). Support for children with developmental disabilities in full inclusion classrooms through self-management. *Journal of Positive Behavioral Interventions, 1*(1), 26–34.

Kreidler, M., (1996). *The evaluation of the pre/post treatment protocol of the PCP*. Unpublished manuscript.

Kurzweil study skills guide, and teaching the language arts tutorial spectronics. (2006). www.spectronicsinoz.com

Lavoie, R. (2005). *It's so much work being your friend: Helping children with learning disabilities find social success*. Atria Books.

Levine, M. (2002). *Educational care* (2nd ed.). Cambridge, MA: Educators Publishing Service.

Lewis, J. *NLDline*. http://www.nldline.com/

Lindamood-Bell drawing with language. www.lblp.com

Lindamood-Bell Visualizing and Verbalizing® program (V/V®). www.lblp.com

Lipton, M., & Nowicki, S. (2009). The social emotional learning framework (SELF): A guide for understanding brain-based social emotional learning impairments. *The Journal of Developmental Processes, 4*, 99–115. https://doi.org/10.1037/a0033435

Loftin, R. L., Gibb, A. C., & Skiba, R. (2005). Using self-monitoring strategies to address behavior and academic issues. *Impact, 18*(2), 12–13.

Lowndes, L. (2003). *How to talk to anyone: 92 little tricks for big success*. McGraw-Hill Education.

Martin, M. (2007). *Helping children with nonverbal learning disabilities to flourish*. London: Jessica Kingsley.
Martinet, J. (2006). *The art of mingling*. St. Martin's Griffin.
Mathmagics. See: https://apps.apple.com/us/app/mathemagics-mental-math/id306586847
McAfee, J. (2013). *Navigating the social world a curriculum for individuals with Asperger's syndrome, high functioning autism and related disorders*. Future Horizon.
McManmon, M.. *College internship program- Michael McManmon*. www.Collegeinternshipprogram.com
Modmath. http://www.modmath.com
National Lekotek Center. www.lekotek.org
Neff, Neff-Lippman and Stockdale. (2002). *The source for visual spatial disorders*. East Moline, IL: LinguiSystems.
Nowicki & Duke. (1992). *Helping the child who doesn't fit in*. Atlanta: Peachtree Publishers
Olsen, J. *Handwriting without tears*. www.hwtears.com
Palombo, J. (2001). *Learning disorders and disorders of the self in children and adolescents*. New York: W. W. Norton & Company.
Palombo, J. (2006). *Nonverbal learning disabilities: A clinical perspective*. New York: W.W. Norton.
Rosner, J. (1979). *Helping children overcome learning difficulties*. New York: Walker.
Rourke, B. P. (1995). The NLD syndrome and the white matter model. In B. P. Rourke (Ed.), *Syndrome of nonverbal learning disabilities: Neurodevelopmental manifestations* (pp. 1–27). New York: Guilford Press.
Rourke, B. P., & Tsatsanis, K. D. (1996). Syndrome of nonverbal learning disabilities: Psycholinguistic assets and deficits. *Topics in Language Disorders, 16*(2), 30–44. https://doi.org/10.1097/00011363-199602000-00005
RULER Program. Yale Center for Emotional Intelligence.
Sala, G., Hooley, M. & Stokes, M. A. (2020). Romantic Intimacy in Autism: A Qualitative Analysis. J Autism Dev Disord. https://doi.org/10.1007/s10803-020-04377-8
Samuelson. *Beth SOS skills for success*. www.sos4students.com
Schloerb, A. P. (2005). The impact of nonverbal Learning disabilities on early development. *Praxis, 5*, 55–60.
Sedgewick, F., Hill, V., & Pellicano, E. (2018). Parent perspectives on autistic girls' friendships and futures. Autism & Developmental Language Impairments. https://doi.org/10.1177/2396941518794497
Semrud-Clikeman, M., Fine, J. G., & Bledsoe, J. (2010). Meta-analysis of empirical literature on NVLD. Paper presented at the International Neuropsychological Society.
Semrud-Clikeman, M., Fine, J. G., & Bledsoe, J. (2015). Social functioning using direct and indirect measures with children with high functioning autism, nonverbal learning disability, and typically developing children. *Child Neuropsychology*, 1–18. https://doi.org/10.1080/09297049.2014.994487
Semrud-Clikeman, M., & Schaefer, V. (2000). Social competence in developmental disorders. *Journal of Psychotherapy in Independent Practice, 4*, 3–20. https://doi.org/10.1300/J288v01n04_01
Semrud-Clikeman, M., & Schafer, V. (2000). Social and emotional competence in children with ADHD and/or learning disabilities. *Journal of Psychotherapy in Independent Practice, 1*(4), 3–19. https://doi.org/10.1300/J288v01n04_02
SimpleMind+- https://simplemind.eu
Stahl, S. (1999). *Vocabulary development*. Cambridge, UK: University Press.
StoryBuilder. https://www.story2.com/blog/storybuilder-storytelling-coach-software
Teaching-Facial-Expressions-of-Emotion.pdf
The grotto grip. www.grottogrip.com
The learning window. www.arkinst.org
Thinking Publications (Social Star) at www.thinkingpublications.com

Thompson, S. (1997). *The source for nonverbal learning disorders*. East Moline, IL: Linguisystems.
Tuley and Bell. (1997). *On Cloud Nine®*. www.lblp.com
Type to learn. https://www.typetolearn.app
Winne, M. *Michelle Garcia winner– Center for social thinking*. www.socialthinking.com
Worlng, D. E., Humphries, T., & Tannock, R. (1999). Spatial and emotional aspects of language inferencing in nonverbal learning disabilities. *Brain and Language, 70*, 220–239.

Chapter 16
Conclusions

In this book we have offered our suggestions for the most current best practices for treating children or adults with NVLD. We hope you have come to appreciate that patients have challenges in multiple areas. Each of them presents with a unique pattern of strengths and weaknesses. We have suggested how to test to determine if your patient meets the criteria for NVLD and how to read and use a test report. You will need to form a team with your patients, their families, schools and tutors, and the many professionals they will meet along their path.

We believe that sharing a transparent, psychologically minded approach offers the best chance of success. In our clinical experience, children/adults face lifelong challenges so we have shared how one needs to think about and plan for these challenges in ways to ensure continued support until it's no longer requested.

In closing, we want to address what success means or will look like. Success doesn't mean that patients will "get over" having NVLD. They do not usually stop having challenges. As there are with all of us, there may be a variety of times in the developmental life cycle when patients will want help, even after interventions and individualized skills have been mastered, as situations change and they develop.

Someone with NVLD can absolutely be successful in their chosen areas with the right continued support. What is important to understand and convey to them is that the need for continued support is not a weakness, but rather an effect of having an "invisible" disability in a neurotypically focused society. Society has expectations and requirements that people with NVLD have difficulties adapting to, so the need for support may be ongoing in order to help your patients adapt to and function in a constantly changing society. This is not a result of personal failings or insufficient therapy or interventions; it is simply an unfortunate side effect of being outside the narrow norm with only limited abilities to change the environment in which they operate. It is similar in some ways to the experience of those with physical disabilities like vision and hearing impairment or mobility issues.

J. Broitman et al., *NVLD and Developmental Visual-Spatial Disorder in Children*, https://doi.org/10.1007/978-3-030-56108-6_16

In Brett's words: "I will not ever be able to stop and say 'okay, here we are, this is the day that the work was preparing me for.' I will always have a learning disability, and it will always keep me from fitting into any kind of normative category. I will continue to encounter people who don't understand my disability, but I have reached a place internally where it is okay with me to not always be perfectly understood. When it matters I will make whatever needs to be known made known, but I think that continuing to be an adult in the process requires that I pick and choose which battles to fight, as you really can't win them all. I have finally reached a place where I can say that I have overcome enough to decide what to overcome next and what to let go. I think that once the next step is no longer clear, you will know that you have really accomplished something". To learn more about Brett's experiences, see Mills, Brett, *"Dealing with NVLD: A family's perspective"* in Broitman, J, Davis, J.M. (ed.) *Treating NVLD in Children: Professional Collaborations for Positive Outcomes.* Chapter 16 New York: Springer (2013).

Gregory, another of our patients, was a practicing lawyer when he finally got diagnosed with NVLD at age 30. He was extremely bright and had used his superior verbal skills to make it through, although at a cost. Not knowing what he was doing wrong or why he didn't fit in had confused and plagued him. His eventual diagnosis helped him figure out what he hated about his law work. He was in contract law and constantly had to produce briefs. While he was brilliant and understood what they said, every single one of them required different "rules" and a different way of writing them up and interpreting them. He realized that he couldn't stand the inconsistencies and had a hard time with the editing process because it wasn't logical. He couldn't easily see the issues and details, which was an absolute requirement in that particular form of law. All of his bosses would say that he wasn't being careful enough in his work, but in reality, he truly couldn't see the problems in his work. His realization enabled him to shift his field of work into one that better suited his neurological makeup; he found an area of specialty that had fewer deadlines and more consistent structure and played more to his verbal strengths. Today he is a much happier man.

Thankfully there are signs that the world is changing and expanding its capacity to accommodate differences in many areas. Advocacy groups have achieved some success in reducing some of the physical barriers and challenges that people with physical disabilities face, increasing accessibility by adding railings, ramps, hearing aid loops, and verbal signage. A recent and more relevant example of increasing societal sensitivity and awareness occurred during the coronavirus pandemic. Britain included people on the autism spectrum as a vulnerable population entitled to special assistance, acknowledging the need for "increased impact of virus" mitigation efforts due to the uncertainties and shifts introduced into their routines.

The evolving awareness of society is an important change for us all, and as it increases, more barriers will be reduced. What we can successfully try to do now, as we do for all our patients, is help them create fulfilling and rewarding lives. We achieve this by teaching them the individualized tools needed for their personal tool box. We can help them figure out how their unique mind works. We can help them break down their problems into manageable chunks that won't overwhelm them or confound their challenges further. We can listen carefully and help them understand what works for them and what doesn't. We can guide them toward telling their family, friends, partners, and colleagues what they need, in a way that can be heard and respected. We can help them advocate for themselves to protect from becoming overwhelmed or shamed for their neurodiversity. We can teach them to think about what kind of life they want and will work for them. We can point them toward a life where they can find pleasure and passion in their work and play and help them learn how to attain it. They can triumph, and helping them accomplish this is a task well worth undertaking.

Reference

Mills, B. (2013). Chapter 16: Dealing with NVLD: A family's perspective. In J. Broitman & J. M. Davis (Eds.), *Treating NVLD in children: Professional collaborations for positive outcomes*. New York: Springer.

Afterword

I am very pleased and personally touched to have been asked to write the afterword for this inspirational book. I am the founder of The NVLD Project whose primary mission is to achieve the recognition of nonverbal learning disability as a valid disorder in the DSM (Diagnostic Statistical Manual). I was inspired to start this nonprofit by my adult daughter who was diagnosed with nonverbal learning disability at age 5. She is now 28. It is critical to get NVLD recognized because it will ultimately allow this population to get the proper education, treatment, and interventions they need. At this time, this invisible disability makes it extremely difficult to have access to constructive help.

I knew my daughter was different from other children even when she was very young. She did not move like other babies, her balance was not great, and when she started preschool, I became very aware that she was different than her classmates. School started on a playground roof. All the other children engaged immediately in play, and my daughter observed for a little while before participating. Other kids noticed she was different too. When my daughter was 4, I experienced how isolating it can be to be a parent of a differently wired kid with social issues. Sometimes other children did not want to have playdates with her. I tried to partner with the school to improve her experience. Ultimately, I got my daughter evaluated to assess what was going on with her developmentally. She was given the diagnosis of NVLD when she was 5 and so the journey began.

My daughter received help from a neuropsychologist, an occupational and a speech/language therapist. She was very fortunate to be both diagnosed early and receive interventions. Nonetheless, the help she received was limited in part because I could never find the right school for her. The support she received helped her

J. Broitman et al., *NVLD and Developmental Visual-Spatial Disorder in Children*, https://doi.org/10.1007/978-3-030-56108-6

tremendously with academic skills but not having the right educational setting limited her integrating some of what she was learning from the specialists. She thrived academically, but her social, visual–spatial, and executive functioning skills were not commensurate with her aptitude and academic achievement.

School is such a critical experience. It was very disheartening to have no good options. We decided to send her to a general education school setting only because the academics were so important to her, and we could not find a school to address her other needs. Eventually the social piece became highly problematic. In high school, she had no friends at school and was very unhappy. I understood but felt helpless to make it better. I could not provide a peer group from which she could learn and grow. We were all lonely but it was she who was suffering the most. I wish I could have created the right school for her. However, I failed in that department.

We tried other interventions, but it was clear that no one really understood her difficulties in a way that helped her to compensate successfully for her deficits. I knew she was not alone and felt something should be done about this population. They deserved to be recognized, helped, and get a proper education. Where to start? I had no clue and so began my journey of talking to educators, therapists, psychologists, and psychiatrists. Initially, I proposed a program to a special education school about instituting a program that focused on social issues, executive functioning, and enrichment. The program was approved and implemented, but it was more geared toward enrichment. It was a great after-school initiative but not what I thought would be most beneficial for this population. I was stymied but determined.

Eventually and fortunately, I met researchers in the Division of Child and Adolescent Psychiatry at Columbia University Irving Medical Center who were very interested in NVLD. My close partnership with one of the authors of this book, Dr. Amy Margolis, was pivotal. I worked closely with Amy to develop a vision and mission for the The NVLD Project. We discussed the issues surrounding this disorder and a light bulb went off. I could potentially help the most people with NVLD if I could fund research that would identify the brain basis of NVLD, provide immediate support to families and educators by developing workshops that could be presented in schools and clinics, and ultimately support randomized clinical trials of interventions for NVLD. All of this work was conceived in support of the ultimate dream: to have NVLD recognized as a valid diagnosis in the DSM.

Through these close collaborations not only did I discover the main mission of The NVLD Project, but I also developed a partnership with the Division of Child and Adolescent Psychiatry at Columbia University Irving Medical Center. I knew it would take many people to help, and fortunately, I have found amazing researchers at Columbia who have been working with my organization since 2012. I am so proud of our accomplishments to date and look forward to achieving even more successes together. It gives me great pleasure to know that the authors of this book met through their involvement with the Advisory Board of the The NVLD Project. In addition to funding research, the The NVLD Project has created a community both for individuals with NVLD who need community so very much and for scientists and practitioners to find one another and further the mission through skillful collaboration. I am so grateful to be a part of this initiative working toward identification of the disorder, treatment, and the educational needs of this population. When it comes to NVLD, it truly does take a village.

Laura Lemle, PhD, Founder and Chairperson
The NVLD Project (212) 257-4828

NVLD PROJECT
COUNT ME IN

www.nvld.org

Appendices

Appendix 1: Proposed New Definition for NVLD: *Developmental Visual–Spatial Disorder*

Created by a consortium led by Prudence W. Fisher, PhD, Division of Child and Adolescent Psychiatry, Columbia University College of Physicians and Surgeons; Dr. Amy Margolis and other Columbia University faculty; NVLD global experts; Drs. Jessica Broitman, Joseph Casey, Jack M. Davis, Jodene Goldenring Fine, Irene Mammarella, M. Douglas Ris, and Margaret Semrud-Clikeman; and members of The NVLD Project's Board of Directors and Advisory Board

Developmental Visual–Spatial Disorder
(Previously Nonverbal Learning Disability)

A. Persistent deficits in processing and integrating visual and spatial information in the presence of developmentally adequate verbal communication skills. The deficits negatively impact directly on social or academic/occupational activities and are manifested by problems in at least four of the following areas, currently or by history (examples are illustrative, not exhaustive; see text):
   Visuospatial awareness (e.g., awareness of own body in space or personal space of others, orienting to new environments)
   Visuospatial construction (e.g., copying visually presented material, planning, orienting, or organizing stimuli that are visual-spatial in nature, drawing, assembling objects)
   Visuospatial memory (e.g., remembering patterns and designs, recalling layout of environments, holding spatial information in mind while simultaneously acting on that information)
   Visuospatial scanning/tracking (e.g., finding information on a page/poster/screen, etc. when there are a lot of distracting images or text, locating things in the presence of clutter, maneuvering in places or situations where other people or things are moving around quickly and in different directions)

J. Broitman et al., *NVLD and Developmental Visual-Spatial Disorder in Children*, https://doi.org/10.1007/978-3-030-56108-6

Spatial estimation (e.g., judging distance, quantity, or time, appropriately using the space on a page, allowing enough time to cross a street when traffic is coming)

Three-dimensional thinking (e.g., imagining how things will look when rotated, route finding, following directions to a location)

Interpreting information presented pictorially (e.g., diagrams, maps, figures, graphs, analog clocks)

B. The visual–spatial deficits were present in the early developmental period but may not have become fully manifest until academic or social demands exceed limited capacities, or may be masked by good verbal strategies or, later in life, by learned strategies.
C. The visual–spatial deficits cause clinically significant distress in the individual or impairment in social, academic, occupational, or other important areas of functioning.
D. The visual–spatial deficits are not better explained by intellectual disability (intellectual developmental disorder) or global developmental delay and are not attributable to uncorrected visual acuity.

Note: Developmental visual–spatial disorder can be diagnosed in addition to the diagnosis of autism spectrum disorder, social (pragmatic) communication disorder, attention deficit hyperactivity disorder, specific learning disorder, or developmental coordination disorder or another mental disorder if the individual meets criteria A through C.

Specify if:

Associated with a known medical or genetic condition or environmental factor (Coding note: Use additional code(s) to identify the associated medical or genetic condition.)

Associated with another neurodevelopmental, mental, or behavioral disorder (Coding note: Use additional code(s) to identify the associated neurodevelopmental, mental, or behavioral disorder(s).)

With or without impairment in social relationships

Note: The diagnostic criteria are to be met based on a clinical synthesis of the individual's history (developmental, medical, family, educational), school reports, and psychoeducational or neuropsychological assessment.

Appendix 2: Intake Form

CHILD Personal Data Form

DATE:_______________ CODE #:______

CHILD'S
NAME:____
____

Last First Middle

ADDRESS:____
____

Street City Zip

HOME PHONE: ____________________

CHILD'S DATE OF BIRTH: ________ AGE:_____ SEX: ___ PLACE OF
BIRTH:_________________

1. PRIMARY CAREGIVER:

____
____

Last First Middle
Relationship to child

ADDRESS:

____
______

(If different than above.)

HOME PHONE: _________________ WORK PHONE: __________________
CELL:________________

EMAIL ADDRESS: ____________________________

EMPLOYER: _________________________________ Number of years at current or
last job:

OCCUPATION: _______________________MONTHLY INCOME:

2. SECONDARY CAREGIVER:

____
____

Last First Middle
Relationship to child

ADDRESS:

____
______

(If different than above.)

HOME PHONE: __________________ WORK PHONE: __________________ CELL:
____

EMAIL ADDRESS:_______________________________

EMPLOYER: ___________________________________ Number of years at last or current job: ________

OCCUPATION: _________________________MONTHLY INCOME:____________________

EDUCATION OF CAREGIVERS: (Highest degree or number of years completed for both.)

____
____

CAREGIVER'S RELATIONSHIP STATUS: (Circle) Married; Separated; Divorced; Domestic Partner; Other (Please explain):

____
____

Length of time in current relationship:

____

Number of prior marriages/domestic partnerships:

____

CHILD'S ETHNICITY: (Circle all that apply) Caucasian, Asian, Hispanic/Latino, Native American, Pacific Islander.
Other:____
__

PARENT'S ETHNICITY: (Circle all that apply) Caucasian, Asian, Hispanic/Latino, Native American, Pacific Islander.
Other:____
_

CHILD'S RELIGIOUS AFFILIATION: (Circle) Protestant; Catholic; Jewish; Islamic; Buddhist; Agnostic; Atheist; Other:

____

PARENT'S RELIGIOUS AFFILIATION: (Circle) Protestant; Catholic; Jewish; Islamic; Buddhist; Agnostic; Atheist; Other:

____

CHILD'S CURRENT LIVING SITUATION:

CHILD'S SIBLINGS: (Include step-siblings and half-siblings and their ages – *in birth order.*) __________

____

____

CURRENT HOUSEHOLD CONSISTS OF:

Name	Relationship to child	Gender	Age
1.) ______________;	______________;	__________;	__________
2.) ______________;	______________;	__________;	__________
3.) ______________;	______________;	__________;	__________
4.) ______________;	______________;	__________;	__________
5.) ______________;	______________;	__________;	__________

VISITATION AND JOINT CUSTODY DETAILS: (Please briefly describe details of child's visitation patterns if applicable.)

____

____

____

CHILD'S EDUCATION HISTORY:

Current Grade Level: _______________

Current
School:____
____

Name Address Phone

Schools Attended since Kindergarten (Names &
Grades):____
____
____

Academic Strengths:
____

Academic Challenges:
____

Extracurricular Interests/Activities:
____

Quality of relationships with peers (Circle): Very good; Good; Uncertain; Poor; Very
Poor.

Describe:
____
_

Briefly describe any challenges making friends:
____

Quality of relationships with teachers (Circle): Very good; Good; Uncertain; Poor; Very
Poor.

Describe:
____
_

Briefly describe any difficulty with attendance or participation in school:
____
____
____

Has your child been placed in special education programs currently or in the past? Yes
_____ No _____

Category____
____

____ Learning Disability (LD):
Subjects____

____ Language Disorder:
Type____

____ Tutoring:
Subjects____
____

CHILD'S MEDICAL HISTORY:

CHILD'S DOCTOR:

____

Name Address Phone

BIRTH & DEVELOPMENT HISTORY:

Pregnancy – length in months: ________

Any illnesses or complications while pregnant? Yes _____ No _____

If yes, please explain briefly:

____

Any substances used during pregnancy: (Circle) Cigarettes; Alcohol; or Drugs.

Please describe use:

____

Biological father's use during conception: (Circle) Cigarettes; Alcohol; or Drugs.

Please describe use:

____

LABOR AND DELIVERY:

Was your child's birth "normal?" Yes _____ No _____

If no, please explain briefly:

____

Birth weight: _______ Length _______

Did mother or baby stay in Special or Intensive Care: Yes _____ No _____

Please describe any problems:

____

____
____

____
____

Please list any birth defects:

____

INFANCY AND EARLY CHILDHOOD (to age 3):

Please rate your child on the following behaviors: Circle 1 if the behavior on the left was present the majority of the time. Circle 5 if the behavior on the right was present the majority of the time. Stages in between are represented by 2, 3, and 4. If there are two behaviors listed, please check which were present if applicable.

quiet and content	1	2	3	4	5
colicky and irritable	1	2	3	4	5
very easy to feed	1	2	3	4	5
daily feeding problems	1	2	3	4	5
slept well	1	2	3	4	5
frequent sleeping problems	1	2	3	4	5
usually relaxed	1	2	3	4	5
often restless	1	2	3	4	5
underactive	1	2	3	4	5
overactive	1	2	3	4	5
cuddly, easy to hold	1	2	3	4	5
did not enjoy cuddling	1	2	3	4	5
easily calmed down	1	2	3	4	5
tantrums	1	2	3	4	5
head-banging	1	2	3	4	5
cautious and careful	1	2	3	4	5
accident prone	1	2	3	4	5
daredevil	1	2	3	4	5
coordinated	1	2	3	4	5
uncoordinated	1	2	3	4	5
enjoyed eye contact	1	2	3	4	5
avoided eye contact	1	2	3	4	5
liked people	1	2	3	4	5
disliked contact with people	1	2	3	4	5

Other problems or comments regarding infancy or early childhood development: ______________________

____
____

____
____

Did any event, health condition, separation, etc., disturb early infant/mother bonding or the developing toddler/mother relationship? Yes _____ No _____

If yes, please explain:

____

____
____

Please describe your child as an infant (temperament, personality, sociability, etc.): _____________________

____
____

MEDICAL EMERGENCIES:

Has your child been taken to the emergency room with a serious emergency, hospitalized, or had outpatient surgery since birth? Yes _____ No _____

If yes, please describe condition/injury, treatment, any surgery, when, how long, and where:_____________

____
____

____
____

If your child ever had a head injury, did he or she lose consciousness?

Yes _____ No _____ How long? ___________________________

Do you see your child as being:

_____ Hyperactive; _____Inattentive; _____ a behavior problem? (Check any that apply.)

Does your child seem to be able to control his or her behavior and attention? Yes _____ No _____

If no, please explain/describe briefly: ____

____

Has your child ever been diagnosed by a psychologist, psychiatrist, or physician, as having ADHD (Attention-Deficit/Hyperactive Disorder)? Yes _____ No _____

If yes, explain briefly: (Include doctor's name, approx. date of testing, medication prescribed, child's response to meds, current status of problem, etc.) ____

____

Please describe any other special health considerations and their treatments, including medications currently being taken by your child: ____

____

Last vision test: ____________________ Results: ____________________

Last hearing test: ____________________ Results: ____________________

CHILD'S CURRENT OVERALL HEALTH:

Excellent _____ Good _____ Fair _____ Poor _____

BEHAVIORAL AND MENTAL HEALTH HISTORY:

Please describe any behaviors that are particularly concerning to you or others: ______________________

____

____

PRIOR MENTAL HEALTH TREATMENT

Names of previous psychotherapists, social workers, psychiatrists, or hospitals:

1.) ____ Dates: ______________________

2.) ____ Dates: ______________________

3.) ____ Dates: ______________________

FAMILY PSYCHIATRIC HISTORY: (i.e. grandparents, father, mother, adoptive parents, siblings, etc. and type of problem, i.e. depression, anxiety, bipolar, substance abuse, etc.)

Family Member Type of Problem

1.) ______________________________; ____

2.) ______________________________; ____

3.) ______________________________; ____

SIGNIFICANT EVENTS IN CHILD'S LIFE: Please circle and describe any of the flowing that happened prior to or since your child's birth. Briefly detail event and indicate your child's age when it occurred.

Event Age

1.) Parent death ____ _______

2.) Sibling death ____ _______

3.) Physical abuse____ _______

4.) Sexual abuse____ _______

5.) Emotional
abuse____

____

6.)
Neglect____

_____ ________

7.)
Abandonment____

______ ________

8.) Volatile parental relationship

____ ________

9.) Parent's
divorce____

____

10.) Parent's re-
marriage____

____

11.) Immigration (from
where?)____- ________

12.) Parental
disability____

____

13.) Sibling
disability/hospitalization____

____

14.) Poverty or serious financial
distress____ ________

15.)
Other____

_____ ________

PRESENT PERSONALITY AND BEHAVIOR:

Please circle all traits that apply to your child *now*.

Happy Moody Friendly Independent Irritable
Sensitive Affectionate Dependent Hard to discipline
Leader Quiet Cooperative Overactive
Tantrums Sad
Follower Prefers to be alone Too responsible Lethargic
Trouble sleeping

CHILD'S SUBSTANCE USE (if applicable):

Please describe your *direct* knowledge of your child's use of the following substances. Include frequency of consumption if known and any problems arising from use:

Alcohol ____

Marijuana ____

Cocaine____

Hallucinogens (LSD, Ecstasy, 'Shrooms, etc.)________________________________

Amphetamines____

Other____

DESCRIPTION OF CURRENT PROBLEM(S):

Reason(s) for seeking child therapy at this time. (Please list your child's problems in order of their concern for you or him/her. If problems involve others, please state their relationship to your child.)

1.) ____

2.) ____

3.) ____

OTHER QUESTIONS:

To your knowledge has your child ever felt like harming himself/herself? Yes _____ No _____

If yes, when?: Month _______ Year _______

Did they act on those feelings? (Please describe.)

____

____

____

What action was taken? (Please describe.)

____

____

____

YOUR RATING OF CHILD'S CURRENT PROBLEM(S):

The pain and distress caused to the family by child's current problem(s) are: (circle the number)

very mild	mild	moderate	severe	very severe
1	2	3	4	5

The likelihood that my child's problem(s) will be solved in the near future is: (circle the number)

Very good	good	uncertain	poor	very poor
1	2	3	4	5

OUTCOME YOU AND/OR CHILD SEEK FROM THERAPY:

I hope that therapy will help my child to: (circle *all* that apply)

Reduce stress	Resolve problems	Learn to live with their problems	Personal Growth	Exploration and greater understanding	Unsure

At the end of therapy, I expect my child's problems to be: (circle the number)

Completely resolved	Mostly resolved	Well on the way to being resolved	Explored but not resolved	Still Unresolved
1	2	3	4	5

Appendix 3: Children's Nonverbal Learning Disabilities Scale

1. Motor Skills

a. My child has problems with balance (e.g. never learned to ride a bike).

Never/Rarely ___Sometimes ___Often/Always ___ I don't know ___

b. My child displays impaired fine motor skills (e.g. significant difficulties learning to tie shoes).

Never/Rarely _Sometimes ___ Often/Always __ I don't know ___

c. My child has problems writing or extremely slow writing.

Never/Rarely __Sometimes ___Often/Always ___ I don't know ___

d. My child seems unusually clumsy.

Never/Rarely ___ Sometimes ___ Often/Always ___ I don't know ___

2. Visual-Spatial Skills

a. My child has difficulty remembering and organizing visual or spatial information (e.g. has difficulty lining up numbers to do a math problem or lining up words neatly on a page).

Never/Rarely ___Sometimes ___Often/Always ___I don't know___

b. My child appears disoriented, lost, or confused when entering a new situation.

Never/Rarely ___Sometimes ___Often/Always ___I don't know ___

c. My child is slow to become familiar with new physical locations (e.g. continues to appear lost or disoriented after repeated exposures to the same location).

Never/Rarely __Sometimes ___Often/Always __I don't know ___

d. My child has difficulty remembering the faces of people they have met.

Never/Rarely __Sometimes ___Often/Always __I don't know ___

e. My child has an auditory memory like a tape recorder.

Yes ____ No ____ I don't know ____

f. My child loses his or her way and needs help finding his or her way around.

Never/Rarely ___Sometimes ___Often/Always ___ I don't know ___

g. My child has unusually strong verbal skills (e.g. an impressive vocabulary or early speech).

Yes ____ No ____ I don't know ____

3. Interpersonal Skills

a. My child often does not get the humor in a joke because they interprets everything so literally.

Never/Rarely ___Sometimes ___Often/Always ___ I don't know ___

b. When interacting with others my child has difficulty reading the other person's non-verbal cues, such as tone of voice or facial expression.

Never/Rarely ___Sometimes ___ Often/Always ___I don't know ___

c. My child interprets what I say very literally (for example, if I tell my child 'to pick themselves up by his or her bootstraps', they appear confused).

Never/Rarely ___Sometimes __Often/Always ___ I don't know ___

d. My child has difficulty transferring what they learns in one social situation to similar social situations. For e.g. my child appears confused when confronted with slight changes in a frequently encountered social situation.

Never/Rarely __Sometimes ___Often/Always __I don't know

The Children's Nonverbal Learning Disabilities Scale© was excerpted, with permission from the author, from the Developmental Screening and Referral Inventory (DSRI) by David B. Goldstein, PhD, 1999.

Guidelines for Scoring the Children's Nonverbal Learning Disabilities Scale

The syndrome of NLD includes a number of specific symptoms. Rourke (1995) has organized these into three primary areas: neuropsychological deficits, academic deficits, and social emotional/adaptational deficits. Neuropsychological deficits include difficulties with tactile and visual perception, psychomotor coordination, tactile and visual attention, nonverbal memory, reasoning, executive functions, and specific aspects of speech and language. Deficits in mathematical reasoning, math calculations, reading comprehension, specific aspects of written language, and handwriting are primary academic concerns. Deficits in social expertise include problems with social cognition and perception as well as difficulties in social interaction.

Some of the symptoms identified with nonverbal learning disabilities are similar to those described for other disorders. Individuals with right hemisphere dysfunction, Asperger's syndrome, and sensory–motor deficiencies each possess a number of characteristics that overlap with those of a nonverbal learning disability. An evaluation by a neuropsychologist can often assist in differential diagnosis.

This is a checklist of characteristics that may be indicative of a nonverbal learning disability. A referral for a more detailed evaluation by a pediatric neuropsychologist to rule in or rule out a NLD requires that the parent report symptoms in all three spheres noted: deficiencies in motor skills, visual–spatial skills, and interpersonal skills.

A referral to a neuropsychologist or for a more in-depth evaluation of a NLD should be considered if the teacher/parent reports deficits "Sometimes" or "Often" on over half the items examining motor skills (at least 3 of the 4 items), visual–spatial skills (at least 4 of the 7 items), and interpersonal skills (at least 3 or the 4 items).

References

Rourke, B. P. (1994). Neuropsychological assessment of children with learning disabilities: Measurement issues. In G. Reid Lyons (Ed.), *Frames of Reference for the Assessment of Learning Disabilities: New Views on Measurement Issues.* Baltimore: Paul H. Brooks.

The Children's Nonverbal Learning Disabilities Scale from the Developmental Screening and Referral Inventory by David B. Goldstein, Ph.D., 1999.

Appendix 4: Developmental Visual–Spatial Disorder Checklist

(Nonverbal Learning Disability)

(Broitman, Margolis, and Davis, 2020)

A developmental visual–spatial disorder (NVLD) has persistent deficits in processing and integrating visual and spatial information in the presence of developmentally adequate verbal communication skills. The deficits negatively impact directly on social or academic/occupational activities and are manifested by problems in at least *four* of the following areas, currently or by history. Endorse with a check all that are present.

Visuospatial awareness, e.g.:

1. Awareness of own body in space or personal space of others, ____
2. Orienting to new environments____________________

Visuospatial construction

1. Copying visually presented material__________
2. Planning, orienting, or organizing stimuli that are visual–spatial in nature, ________
3. Drawing, ________________
4. Assembling objects____________________

Visuospatial memory

1. Remembering patterns and designs,_____________
2. Recalling layout of environments,___________________
3. Holding spatial information in mind while simultaneously acting on that information______________________________

Visuospatial scanning / tracking, e.g.:

1. Finding information on a page/poster/screen, etc. when there are a lot of distracting images or text, __________________
2. Locating things in the presence of clutter and maneuvering in places or situations where other people or things are moving around quickly and in different directions______________________

Spatial estimation, e.g.:
1. Judging distance ____________________
2 Quantity or time________________________
3. Appropriately using the space on a page______________
4. Allowing enough time to cross a street when traffic is coming_______
Three-dimensional thinking
1. Imagining how things will look when rotated______________
2. Route finding and following directions to a location____________
Interpreting information presented pictorially
1. Diagrams___________________________________
2. Maps___________________________________
3. Figures_________________________________
3. Graphs___________________________________
4 Analog clocks_______________________________

Appendix 5: Scale of Executive Function

Peggy Hock and Jane McClure © 2008
Student: ______________________ Birthdate: ________
Gender: M F Today's Date: ____________
Completed by (circle one): Student Parent Tutor Resource teacher Name: ______________________

Instructions: The following are areas in which the student may be receiving assistance at home and at school. For each item, indicate the level of independence the student has demonstrated over the past 2 months.

	Always	Most of the time	Sometimes	Rarely	Never
Sleep:					
Independently goes to bed at appropriate time					
Independently wakes up and gets up on time					
Personal hygiene:					
Bathes and washes hair regularly without reminders					
Combs hair, brushes teeth, and shaves without reminders					
Independently chooses appropriate attire for each day's weather and activities					
Independently remembers to take prescribed medications					
Nutrition:					
Can prepare simple breakfast, lunch, and snacks					
Independently makes good food choices					
Independently schedules meals appropriately					

	Always	Most of the time	Sometimes	Rarely	Never
Time management:					
Appropriately limits use of electronic media (computer, TV, games, cell phone)					
Independently schedules time for homework and follows through					
Independently keeps track of daily assignments					
Independently plans steps to complete projects					
Independently plans time for step-by -step completion of projects					
Turns in long-term projects/assignments on time					
Feels confident of own ability to schedule and handle school assignments and chores					
Organization:					
Independently turns completed homework to teachers on time					
Independently brings home or plans to obtain materials required to complete homework (textbooks, assignment sheets, art supplies, etc.)					
Reliably brings home announcements, etc. from school					
Reliably returns completed forms, etc. to school					
Keeps track of personal items at school					
Independently locates personal items at home					
Independently maintains orderly backpack and binder					

	Always	Most of the time	Sometimes	Rarely	Never
Money management:					
Can create workable a budget for personal expenses					
Can manage daily personal expenses within a budget					
Can independently balance a checkbook					
Reading:					
Understands content of textbook material at first reading					
Can take notes from written material, identifying main ideas and supporting points					
Can retain information obtained from reading					
Reads for pleasure					
Writing:					
Can organize own ideas for writing					
Uses correct grammar when writing					
Uses correct spelling (or spell check) when writing					

	Always	Most of the time	Sometimes	Rarely	Never
Can independently write a 3–5-page research paper					
Note taking:					
Understands information presented orally					
Can stay focused and listen for an entire class period					
Can listen, take notes, and identify key points and supporting ideas					
Can learn new material by reviewing own notes					
Can accurately copy notes from board or screen					
Test taking:					
Can effectively demonstrate acquired knowledge on each of the following:					
Multiple-choice test					
Short answer test					
Fill-in-the-blank test					
Essay test					
True/false test					
Student currently uses the following academic accommodations:					
Assistive technology for reading (cf Kurzweil)					
Preferential seating					
Reduced homework					
Quiet testing environment					
Up to 50% extra time on tests					
Reader for tests					
Use of a computer for all written assignments					
Use of computer for tests					
Scribe for tests					
Alternative test format					

Indicate any additional support student receives for activities of school or daily living.

Appendix 6: The SVS Questionnaire

(Cornoldi et al. 2003)

Shortened Visuospatial Questionnaire for Teachers

Items followed by "VSLD" are used for obtaining the VSLD score.

(1 = not at all, 2 = sometimes, 3 = most of the time, 4 = completely)

1. Can the child easily memorize material such as names, information, and poems?
1 2 3 4
2. Is the child able to make use of the available space when drawing? VSLD
1 2 3 4
3. Can the child use tools such as scissors, set square, and ruler, which require independent and coordinated use of both hands? VSLD
1 2 3 4
4. Does the child understand spoken commands or texts, which involve spatial relationships? VSLD
1 2 3 4
5. Is the child able to execute complex everyday movements (e.g., tying shoelaces)? VSLD
1 2 3 4
6. Does the child show a good understanding of spatial relationships in calculation, and can he or she write numbers in a column correctly? VSLD
1 2 3 4
7. Does the child have good spatial orientation abilities? VSLD
1 2 3 4
8. Is the child good at drawing? VSLD
1 2 3 4
9. Can the child easily interact with friends?
1 2 3 4
10. Has the child reached a good linguistic learning level for his or her age?
1 2 3 4
11. Has the child reached a good mathematics learning level for his or her age?
1 2 3 4
12. Is the child competent in learning contexts, which rely on visuospatial skills? VSLD
1 2 3 4
13. Is the child distracted easily?
1 2 3 4
14. Is the child often restless and/or hyperactive?
1 2 3 4
15. Is the child a good observer of the environment in which he or she lives? VSLD
1 2 3 4
16. Does the child demonstrate interest in new objects, and can he or she deal with them? VSLD
1 2 3 4
17. Does the child show good overall cognitive potential?
1 2 3 4
18. Does the child have a poor sociocultural background?
1 2 3 4

Appendix 7: The SVS Questionnaire

(Cornoldi et al. 2003)

Shortened Visuospatial Questionnaire for Children

Items followed by "VSLD" are used for obtaining the VSLD score.

(1 = not at all, 2 = sometimes, 3 = most of the time, 4 = completely)

1. I can easily memorize material such as names, information, and poems.

1 2 3 4

2. I like reading.

1 2 3 4

3. I am able to use tools such as scissors, set square, and ruler? VSLD

1 2 3 4

4. I have good spatial orientation abilities (e.g., in a supermarket, I'm able to find the exit easily). VSLD

1 2 3 4

5. I am able to execute complex everyday movements (e.g., tying shoelaces). VSLD

1 2 3 4

6. I am able to write numbers in a column correctly.

1 2 3 4

7. I have good grades in reading.

1 2 3 4

8. My exercise books are orderly.

1 2 3 4

9. I have good grades in mathematics.

1 2 3 4

10. I am easily distracted.

1 2 3 4

11. I am often restless and I am not able to stay seated during lessons.

1 2 3 4

12. When I am standing in line, I remember who is in front of me and who is behind me. VSLD

1 2 3 4

13. When I look at a picture, I am able to recall the details of the image. VSLD

1 2 3 4

14. I should be able to reproduce the exact location of the school desks in my class. VSLD

1 2 3 4

15. It is easy for me to make friends.

1 2 3 4

Appendix 8: Problem Breakdown Checklist

(Melcher and Broitman, 2020)

Problem Break down checklist:

Ask your patient to answer the following questions:

1. Baseline Criteria:

   a. How am I feeling physically?

      Light sensitivity: 0 1 2 3 4

      If above 2, do not attend

      Sound sensitivity: 0 1 2 3 4

      If above 2, do not attend

      Headache 0 1 2 3 4

      Exhaustion: 0 1 2 3 4

      Blood sugar: 0 1 2 3 4

      Hydration: 0 1 2 3 4

      Other: 0 1 2 3 4

   b. How am I feeling emotionally?

      Event related stress:

      Logistical: 0 1 2 3 4

      Content: 0 1 2 3 4

      If at or over 4 between the two categories, do not attend

      Other short-term stress: 0 1 2 3 4

      Long-term stress: 0 1 2 3 4

   c. What is the weather like?

      Temperature:

      Over 25 degrees C

      Under 25 degrees C

      Humidity:

      Over 50%

      Under 50%

d. Logistics:

Length of transportation?

1. Long: over 1 hour
2. Medium: 30-60 minutes
3. Short: under 30 minutes.

Method of transportation?

Train/Subway:

1. New subway: How many transfers?
2. Old subway: How many stops?

<u>If over 5 stops + over 25C + medium OR low importance, do not attend</u>

Bus:

1. How many transfers?
2. How familiar with getting on and getting off points?

f. Cost of participation:

Over $20 (or whatever is with in normal budget)

Under $20

g. Content:

Event type:

Very social (ie pub night/party)

Medium social (ie 1:1 or small group)

Low social (ie performance, cinema)

Event importance:

High: very unique OR professionally important

Medium: moderately unique OR culturally/socially important

Low: not especially unique OR not socially/professionally important

Event duration:

Long: 3+ hours

Medium: 1.5-3 hours

Short: less than 90 minutes

h. Post-event recovery requirements (what are the after effects of attending the event):

1. Social: 0 1 2 3 4
2. Light/heat/humidity: 0 1 2 3 4
3. Sound: 0 1 2 3 4
4. Other: 0 1 2 3 4

Total: /16, if over 8, do not attend

Appendix 9: Diagnosing Environmental Challenges Checklist

(also can be used when breaking down/diagnosing how to deal with an issue)

Do you or does your child have any sensitivities to the following?

Sensory

Light –

Brightness________

Inside vs. outside__________

Colors of light_____________

Screen color/brightness__________________

Heat –

Humidity____________

Sunburn______________

Temperature_________________

Cold____________________

Wind_________________

Sound –

Total amount of noise in various environments______________

Difficulty filtering out noise from multiple sources_____________

Sound sensitivity at different times of day_____________

Shampoo______________

Clothing material____________

Toothbrushing_____________

Hair brushing______________

Clothing collar_____________

Clothing tags______________

Taste –

Mushy_________________

Spicy_________________

Acidic_________________

Mix-up of taste/texture____________________

Color causing foods to require visual separation____________

Dislike of combined textures requiring food separation__________

Social area

Physical aspects of social environments which might include:

Space____________
Size_______________
Light_______________
Noise_____________
Heat________________
Clothing requirements__________________
Nonverbal aspects of social environments which might include:
Levels of structure in activity__________________
Number of known vs. unknown people____________
Number of people total__________________
Purpose of event (familiar vs. unfamiliar) ____________
Addition of food/alcohol________________
Logistical aspects of social environments which might include:
The amount of transit time_______________
Complexity of transit______________
Familiarity of transit _______________
The flexibility of transit/start time__________________
Psychological aspects of social environments which might include:
Innate or trained social anxiety___________________
Outside expectations and perceptions of "should"______

Appendix 10: Sensory Modulation Checklist

(see Sensory-Processing-Disorder.com. Here you can find infant/child/teen and adult versions of this checklist)

Do you or your child have any of the following:

General modulation

_______ Has unusual eating habits (strong preferences, eats at odd times, etc.)

_______ Has unusual sleeping habits or sleep schedule

_______ Has great difficulty with transitions, be they major life changes or small everyday stuff (one activity to another, going from inside to outdoors, etc.)_______ Becomes engrossed in one single activity for a long time and seems to tune out everything else

_______ Spends hours at a time on fantasy or video games and activities_______ Very high or very low energy level

_______ Are resistant to change in daily life and surrounding environment

Over-responsiveness

_______ Bothered by clothes; certain materials, tags, seams, pantyhose, ties, belts, turtlenecks. May have to wear shorts, skirts, or pants exclusively, etc.

_______ Bothered by "light touch"; someone lightly touching/rubbing the hand, face, leg, or back

_______ Excessively ticklish

_______ Distressed by others touching; would rather be the "toucher" than the "touchee." May not like being hugged

_______ Very sensitive to pain, especially as compared to others

_______ Dislikes the feeling of showers or getting splashed

_______ Difficulty going to the beach, as the sand is irritating to the touch

_______ Avoid touching anything "messy"

_______ Washes hands constantly and/or only touches things through fabric or with fingertips

_______ Cannot wear new or "stiff" clothes that have not been washed or soaked in fabric softener_______ Hates to be barefoot or hates to wear shoes and/or socks

_______ Frequently gets car sick, air sick, and motion sick

_______ Difficulty riding on elevators, escalators, or moving sidewalks

_______ Avoids amusement park rides that drop, climb, spin, or go upside down

_______ Difficulty eating foods with mixed textures or one particular texture

_______ Prefers very bland foods, dislikes anything spicy

_______ Become nauseated or gags from certain cooking, cleaning, perfume, public restroom, or bodily odors

_______ Become overstimulated or overaroused when people come to the house or when in crowded places

_______ Overly excited/aroused in group settings

_______ Avoids crowds and hides, disappears, or acts out when guests come over

_______ Sensitive to noises that other people are not bothered by (clocks, refrigerators, fans, people talking, blenders, vacuum cleaners, animals, outdoor construction, etc.)

_______ Easily distracted by auditory or visual stimuli

_______ Cannot attend certain public events or places due to excessive noise

_______ Overreacts to loud noises, like sirens

_______ Can't sleep if room isn't completely dark

_______ Fearful of heights

_______ Bothered by hands or face being dirty

Under-responsiveness

_______ May fail to recognize stimuli that most would find alerting or strong

_______ Unable to identify foods that have gone bad by smell

_______ Difficulty being able to smell dangerous smells (smoke, noxious/hazardous solvents, or something burning in the oven)

_______ Doesn't seem to notice pain; get shots/cuts/bruises and hardly feel a thing

_______ Lethargic, hard to get going, appears "lazy" and unmotivated

_______ Doesn't seem to notice if hands or face is dirty

_______ Is/was a late potty trainer (didn't notice need to go) or has/had chronic bed wetting issues

_______ Doesn't seem to get dizzy

_______ Might not catch self when falling or protect self from getting hurt; lacks reflexes

_______ Doesn't interact with peers or adults; is hard to engage, an observer and not a "doer"

_______ Is the last to notice when a person enters the room, if they notice at all

_______ Difficulty waking up in the morning (may not even notice alarm clock)

Sensory Seeking

_______ Loves to touch and be touched, has to touch everything

_______ Has to fidget and "fiddle" with things all the time; pens, pencils, rubber band, *anything* within reach

_______ Often touches and twists own hair or other's hair

_______ Is a thrill seeker; loves fast and/or dangerous rides and sports

_______ Seeks out fast, spinning, and/or upside down carnival rides

_______ Will often rock or sway body back and forth while seated or standing still

_______ Frequently tip chair on back two legs

_______ Restless when sitting through a lecture, presentation, or movie

_______ Constantly chews on things, sucks thumb, and/or grits teeth

_______ Prefers foods with very strong tastes and flavors

_______ Constantly bites nails or fingers

_______ Bites lips or insides of cheeks

_______ Frequently shakes leg

_______ Loves to sleep under multiple sheets or heavy blankets

_______ Seeks out crashing and "squishing" activities; may jump on furniture or run into other people

_______ Cracks knuckles often

_______ Loves crunchy foods (popcorn, carrots, chips, nuts, pretzels, etc.)

_______ Identifies objects by smell, has to smell everything, uses smell to determine whether or not to like something or someone

_______ Great difficulty settling down for sleep

Sensory Discrimination

_______ Can't identify objects by touch alone

_______ Difficulty finding things in a desk, bag, or pocket without looking

_______ Difficulty heating food to the correct temperature, feeling if it is too hot or too cold

_______ Difficulty locating items in a cupboard, in a drawer, in the closet, or on a grocery shelf

_______ Difficulty with recognizing/interpreting/following traffic signs

_______ Gets disoriented and/or lost easily in stores, buildings, etc.

_______ Difficulty concentrating on or watching a movie/TV show when there is background noise or distractions

_______ Difficulty remembering or understanding what people are saying

_______ Difficulty following directions if given two or three at one time

_______ Cannot complete concentrated tasks if noises present

_______ Talks too loud or too soft

_______ Difficulty licking an ice cream cone neatly

_______ Difficulty with speech and annunciation

_______ Bumps into things frequently

_______ Often pushes too hard on objects, accidentally breaking them
_______ Difficulty judging how much pressure to apply when doing tasks or picking something up
_______ Often reverses numbers and letters or process them backward
_______ Difficulty telling time on an analog clock
_______ Difficulty reading and understanding a map, bus schedule, and directions
_______ Difficulty organizing and grouping things by categories, similarities, and/or differences
_______ Difficulty reading text on computer screens
_______ Difficulty distinguishing different tastes and/or flavors of food and/or drink items
_______ Difficulty lining up numbers correctly for math problems and/or balancing a checkbook

Sensory-Based Motor Abilities

_______ Has difficulty learning to ride a bike or other moving equipment
_______ Clumsy, uncoordinated, and accident-prone
_______ Difficulty walking on uneven surfaces
_______ Difficulty with fine motor tasks, such as buttoning, zipping, tying, playing games with small parts, closing ziplock bags, etc.
_______ Confuses right and left sides
_______ Prefers sedentary tasks, avoiding sports or physical activities
_______ Difficulty with handwriting; hard to read, writes slowly, gets wrist cramps
_______ Frequently bumps into people and things
_______ Easily fatigued with physical tasks
_______ Frequently misses when putting objects on a table
_______ Messy eater, difficulty using eating utensils, spilling and dropping food frequently
_______ Often knocks drinks or other things over when reaching for them
_______ Has difficulty pouring drinks
_______ Frequently drops items
_______ Often hums or talks to self while concentrating on a task
_______ Significant difficulty learning to tie things (shoes, bags, etc.)
_______ Difficulty with motor tasks requiring several steps
_______ Difficulty learning new motor tasks (a new dance, sport or exercise activity, how to drive, etc.)
_______ Loses balance frequently, maybe even when standing still
_______ Significant difficulty learning to type without looking at the keyboard

Social and Emotional

_______ Dislikes changes in plans or routines, needing structure
_______ Often described as "stubborn," "defiant," or "uncooperative"
_______ Is very emotional and sensitive, may also be prone to crying
_______ Can't seem to finish anything
_______ Has difficulty making decisions

_______ Is seen as rigid, bossy, and controlling
_______ Prefers solitary activities over group participation
_______ Is often impatient and/or impulsive
_______ Doesn't always register or understand social cues and nonverbal language
_______ Difficulty with authority figures
_______ Trouble relating to and socializing with peers and colleagues
_______ Has difficulty accepting defeat or forgiving self
_______ Frequently gets angry or has moments of rage
_______ Easily frustrated
_______ Needs sameness and routines; needs to know what to expect
_______ Gets frequent panic or anxiety attacks
_______ Has many fears and/or phobias
_______ OCD-type qualities; can't let foods touch each other on a plate, has to wear clothes a certain way, or other obsessions and compulsions
_______ Is easily distractible and often unorganized
_______ Hates surprises
_______ Difficulty seeking out and maintaining relationships
_______ Avoids eye contact

Internal Regulation

_______ Difficulty falling asleep or getting on a sleep schedule
_______ Heart rate issues, including unnecessary speeding, not slowing down when at rest, or not speeding up for tasks that require a higher heart rate
_______ Respiration too fast or slow for the appropriate state of arousal
_______ Over- or under-sensitive to bowel and bladder sensations
_______ Over- or under-sensitive to the sensations of hunger and thirst
_______ Irregular, inconsistent bowel, bladder, and appetite sensations
_______ Difficulty with temperature regulation of the body

See https://spdsupport.org/resources/files/adolescent-adult-spd-symptom-checklist.pdf

Appendix 11: Blank Brochure from the Brooklyn Learning Center for Child Assessment Report

BROOKLYN LEARNING CENTER

142 Joralemon Street 3E
Brooklyn New York 11201
PHONE 718-935-0400
BrooklynLearningCenter.com

Student: **Feedback Date:**

Big picture:.

Strengths

Challenges

Things for school to provide

Things to keep on doing

Study Strategies

Appendix 12: Key Terms and Definitions

Developmental Coordination Disorder: Also known as developmental dyspraxia. A chronic neurological disorder beginning in childhood that can affect planning of movements and coordination as a result of brain messages not being accurately transmitted to the body. It may be diagnosed in the absence of other motor or sensory impairments like cerebral palsy, muscular dystrophy, multiple sclerosis, or Parkinson's disease.

Dyscalculia: Refers to a wide range of lifelong learning disabilities involving math. Dyscalculia can vary from person to person. There is no single type of math disability. It can include difficulty in learning or comprehending arithmetic, such as difficulty in understanding numbers, learning how to manipulate numbers, and learning facts in mathematics.

Dyslexia: Dyslexia is a learning disorder characterized by difficulty reading due to problems identifying speech sounds and learning how they relate to letters and words.

Dyspraxia: A disorder that affects motor skill development. People with dyspraxia have trouble planning and completing fine motor tasks. This can vary from simple motor tasks such as waving goodbye to more complex tasks like brushing teeth.

Executive Functioning: Refers to neuropsychological functions including decision-making, planning, initiative, assigning priority, sequencing, motor control, emotional regulation, inhibition, problem-solving, planning, impulse control, establishing goals, monitoring results of action, self-correcting.

Nonverbal Learning Disability/Disorder: A neurological disorder or syndrome characterized by a significant discrepancy between higher verbal skills and lower motor and visuospatial skills on IQ and neuropsychological tests. This syndrome includes specific assets and deficits. The assets include early speech and vocabulary development, remarkable rote memory skills, attention to detail, early reading skills development, and excellent spelling skills. Four major categories of deficits and dysfunction also present themselves: motoric (lack of coordination, severe balance problems, and difficulties with graphomotor skills), visual–spatial–organizational social (lack of ability to comprehend nonverbal communication, difficulties adjusting to transitions and novel situations, and deficits in social judgment and social interaction), and sensory (sensitivity in any of the sensory modes: visual, auditory, tactile, taste, or olfactory).

NLD: An abbreviation for nonverbal learning disability/disorder most commonly used on the East Coast of Northern America.

NVLD: An abbreviation for nonverbal learning disability/disorder most commonly used on the West Coast of Northern America.

Pragmatic Language Impairment (PLI): Sometimes known as social (pragmatic) communication disorder (SCD). Impairment in understanding pragmatic areas of language. This type of impairment was previously called semantic–pragmatic disorder (SPD). Individuals with PLI have particular trouble understanding the social meaning of what others are saying, especially idioms and metaphors.

Psychoeducational Evaluation: A written assessment of psychological aspects of learning and academic skills. Evaluations provide estimates of intellectual and cognitive abilities and educational achievement levels. Psychoeducational evaluation yields recommendations for educational planning.

Social Emotional Processing: The ability to comprehend nonverbal communication, adjust to transitions and novel situations, and use social judgment during social interaction.

Specific Learning Disabilities/Disorders: Refers to neurological disorders that can affect acquisition of certain academic, language, and speech skills. Types of learning disabilities include reading (dyslexia), mathematics (dyscalculia), and writing (dysgraphia).

Visual–Spatial Disorders: Includes difficulties with visual imaging, visual recall, faulty spatial perceptions, difficulties with executive functions, and problems with spatial relations.

Index

J. Broitman et al., *NVLD and Developmental Visual-Spatial Disorder in Children*, https://doi.org/10.1007/978-3-030-56108-6

The manufacturer's authorised representative in the EU is Springer Nature Customer Service Centre GmbH, Europaplatz 3, 69115 Heidelberg, Germany. If you have any concerns regarding our products, please contact ProductSafety@springernature.com

Printed and bound by CPI Group (UK) Ltd, Croydon, CR0 4YY
30/09/2026
02225498-0005